WITHOUT COMPASSION,
THERE IS NO HEALTHCARE

Without Compassion, There Is No Healthcare

Leading with Care in a Technological Age

Edited by
BRIAN D. HODGES, GAIL PAECH,
AND JOCELYN BENNETT

McGill-Queen's University Press
Montreal & Kingston • London • Chicago

ISBN 978-0-2280-0376-2 (cloth)
ISBN 978-0-2280-0377-9 (paper)
ISBN 978-0-2280-0461-5 (ePDF)
ISBN 978-0-2280-0462-2 (ePUB)

Legal deposit fourth quarter 2020
Bibliothèque nationale du Québec

Printed in Canada on acid-free paper that is 100% ancient forest free
(100% post-consumer recycled), processed chlorine free

This book has been published with the help of a grant from the Canadian
Federation for the Humanities and Social Sciences, through the Awards to
Scholarly Publications Program, using funds provided by the Social Sciences
and Humanities Research Council of Canada. Funding was also received
from Associated Medical Services.

Funded by the Government of Canada / Financé par le gouvernement du Canada
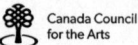
Canada Council for the Arts / Conseil des arts du Canada

We acknowledge the support of the Canada Council for the Arts.

Nous remercions le Conseil des arts du Canada de son soutien.

Library and Archives Canada Cataloguing in Publication

Title: Without compassion, there is no healthcare: compassionate care in a
technological age / edited by Brian D. Hodges, Gail Paech, and Jocelyn Bennett.

Names: Hodges, Brian David, 1964– editor. | Paech, Gail, 1947– editor. | Bennett,
Jocelyn, 1958– editor.

Description: Includes bibliographical references and index.

Identifiers: Canadiana (print) 20200279254 | Canadiana (ebook) 20200279424 |
ISBN 9780228003779 (paper) | ISBN 9780228003762 (cloth) | ISBN
9780228004615 (ePDF) | ISBN 9780228004622 (ePUB)

Subjects: LCSH: Medical technology. | LCSH: Medical care. | LCSH: Compassion.

Classification: LCC R855.3 .W58 2020 | DDC 610—dc23

This book was typeset by Marquis Interscript in 10.5 / 13 Sabon.

The more distracted we become, and the more emphasis we place on speed at the expense of depth, the less likely and able we are to care ...

Being attentive to the needs of others might not be the point of life, but it is the work of life.

Jonathan Safran Foer, "How Not to Be Alone,"
New York Times, 8 June 2013

Contents

Contents

Tables and Figures

A Call to Caring

Brian D. Hodges

As the year 2020 began, the world watched in horror as a virulent virus, now known as COVID-19, spread around the globe. It closed down the economy of almost every country in the world, sickened millions, and proved deadly for older adults and those with serious health conditions. Health professionals rallied, harnessing oxygen and ventilators in overcrowded, under-prepared intensive care units, medical wards, and long-term care facilities. Public health and home and community care prepared to support and manage large numbers of our population at home in self-isolation and quarantine. Healthcare providers also deployed unbelievable compassion for patients, families, and for each other.

In the midst of these heroic demonstrations of compassion, caring, and kindness, models of care shifted seemingly overnight. Relevant to the theme of this book is the incredibly rapid concurrent virtualization of care in the community, clinics, and hospitals of countries affected by the pandemic. In a matter of weeks, headlines on virtual care shifted from "Canada Has Long Way to go on Virtual Care" (Vogel 2020, E227), to "Your Next Visit with a Doctor May Not be Face to Face" (Ogilvie 2020). In my own hospital, which in regular times has over a million ambulatory visits per year, 80 per cent of ambulatory care was shifted online in a matter of two weeks! Understanding both the effectiveness and the patient and family experience of this dizzying systems change will take months, but suffice it to say the digital transformation experienced an enormous jump forward. It is now more urgent than ever to understand what it means that huge swaths of healthcare can be conducted online, at a distance, and mediated by technology.

As this book comes into print, the crisis it not over, and it is likely that COVID-19 will return in further waves. For many healthcare workers it recalls the medical, economic, and psychological devastation unleashed by Severe Acute Respiratory Syndrome (SARS) in 2003, a virus that infected a tiny fraction of the number already touched by COVID-19. The authors here address critical issues that can support learning from this pandemic in a way that we have not learned in the past.

COMPASSION IN HEALTHCARE

Beyond the implementation of virtual care, other technologies are also changing life significantly for those of us who work in or require healthcare. Hospitals have launched patient portals that give instant access to test results and appointments. In clinics, operating rooms, and community settings, computers that employ artificial intelligence (AI) are augmenting the work of human health professionals. It seems every day new technologies bring fantastical advances to care.

The technological transformation underway in healthcare is worthy of particularly focused attention, as unlike other industries (banking, commerce, and transportation) which are all concerned with human experience, healthcare is rooted in something deeper: the very purpose of healthcare work is anchored strongly by compassion – by a commitment to attend to and alleviate the suffering of others. This book illuminates challenges and opportunities that are specific to the future of healthcare. Within an evolving technological landscape, how can healthcare remain grounded in, and driven by, its compassionate purpose?

While the editors and authors of this book hold diverse perspectives, we have worked in concert to develop two premises. First, human compassion must remain central to the means and ends of healthcare work. Second, technologies can and should be aligned with this goal, but that is only possible with vigilant attention to their specific capacities, effects, and potential harms. The ways that humans choose to design, acquire, and employ technologies will determine whether compassionate healthcare is fostered or undermined.

Yet, for some time, compassion has lost prominence as the governing tenet of healthcare work. Compassionate care is vulnerable when stacked against the constant imperative to be efficient, the distancing gaze of science, and the rapid, expansive logic of automation. When compassion is diminished, healthcare becomes ineffective or even harmful to those who receive treatment, as well as for those who provide it. Compassion must first be reaffirmed as a guiding principle at the core of future healthcare systems. It must then be brought to bear upon the technological advances that are fast unfolding. Each chapter in this collection serves one or both of these objectives.

Terms for governing values, such as "compassion," tend to accrue many meanings. This is part of their power and potential as a uniting force, but it can also produce confusion and discourage precision. We must, therefore, be vigilant about what we mean by "compassion." In preparing this book, we began with established definitions as baselines. Following the *Oxford Handbook of Compassion Science*, we mean *empathy* to be "an emotional experience that is the same (or nearly the same) as what another person is feeling or expected to feel" (Seppälä, Simon-Thomas, et al. 2017, 63) and *compassion* to be "sensitivity to the pain or suffering of another, coupled with a deep desire to alleviate that suffering" (Seppälä, Simon-Thomas, et al. 2017, 42). Empathy is necessary but not sufficient for compassion; the latter requires an inclination to act. Contributing authors were encouraged to take these definitions as a point of departure. As scholars of language, however, many of us are aware that the meaning and power of words cannot be readily contained. Some authors have chosen to extend, examine, and challenge these definitions. In particular, each of the first three chapters offers a distinct approach to the concept of *compassion*.

This book imagines a future in which efficiency, science, and automation serve, rather than subsume, the ends of human connection and well-being. Our goals are to help healthcare providers, educators, leaders, and policy-makers understand and anticipate shifts in the healthcare landscape and create healthcare systems that preserve the centrality of compassion. Considered more broadly, healthcare systems provide a window onto larger social and cultural concerns. If the distinctly human experiences of empathy and compassion can be displaced from the core of the "caring professions," they (and we) must certainly be endangered.

"I DON'T CARE"

Dr William (Bill) Shragge was a cardiovascular thoracic surgeon with a gift for teaching and love of clinical care. He shared with me a story that illustrates why the book you are reading needs to exist.

It was late at night. Bill, a surgical fellow in training, was receiving hand-off from a colleague, also a surgical trainee. Bill's colleague told

him about a child patient who needed to go to the operating room
that night for urgent surgery. Bill thanked his colleague for providing
details about the heart vessels and surgical plan. Then he asked, "Can
you tell me something about the child, the child's life or family?" His
colleague responded, "Oh, I don't care about *that*." A spark was lit.
The young Bill Shragge, future surgeon, teacher, and healthcare leader,
promised himself that night that he would work toward a future in
which no health professional could ever say, "I don't care" – a future
in which healthcare never lost its anchor in compassion.

Many years later, Bill became the CEO of Associated Medical
Services (AMS) Healthcare, a Canadian charitable organization that
has been dedicated for more than eighty years to catalyzing change
in healthcare education and practice. Bill worked with healthcare
leaders and educators to create the AMS Phoenix Project: A Call to
Caring. Established in 2011, this initiative was based on the premise
that healthcare professionals do their best work when they balance
the technical and human dimensions of healthcare. Sadly, Bill was
diagnosed with cancer in the early days of the AMS Phoenix Project,
and he died in 2012. On some days during his cancer journey, Bill
would describe having had an amazing experience at the hospital
clinic or with his homecare professionals. This gave him hope about
a healthcare system built on compassion. On other days, however, he
was saddened at the callousness and technocratic approach of his
caregivers, despairing about care that was dehumanized.

THE AMS PHOENIX PROGRAM: GALVANIZING
A COMMUNITY FOR COMPASSION

The Phoenix Project grew into the Phoenix Program in 2016: a five-
year initiative designed to influence healthcare culture such that learning and practice environments balance scientific knowledge with
high-quality person-centred care. Acting as a catalyst for change, AMS
Healthcare supports fellowships and grants that focus on developing
tangible ways to strengthen health professionals' resilience; new curricula to instill knowledge, skills, and values integral to compassionate
care; and innovations to foster healthy, respectful, and collaborative
work environments. They joined with partners across Ontario,
Canada, and around the world to build a critical mass of educators,
healthcare professionals, researchers, and policy-makers focused on
compassion in healthcare.

The AMS Phoenix Program became one of the largest efforts any-where to build community and to marshal arguments and evidence in support of compassionate healthcare. This book brings together many members of that community, drawing upon a large and growing movement of individuals and organizations sharing a commitment to understanding and fostering compassion. The authors reflect the diversity of that community. They work in both urban and rural set-tings. They practice in many different professions and specialties. They are educators, administrators, leaders, policy-makers, learners, and patients. What unites them all is a deep commitment to ensuring that compassion anchors healthcare, particularly at a time when emerging technologies are rapidly changing what healthcare is.

TECHNOLOGY AND THE CALL TO CARING

Rapidly emerging technologies present a new challenge and a burning platform. As I explore in the opening chapter of this book, the disrup-tive combination of machine learning, AI, data analytics, and robotics is coalescing to automate healthcare to an unprecedented degree. Recognizing this challenge, the current AMS Healthcare Board and its CEO Gail Paech have issued a call to action: a call for healthcare professionals, educators, and policy-makers to get out in front of these changes. A call to ensure that technologies are held accountable to healthcare's compassionate purpose. This book issues that call to action and lays a foundation for pursuing it.

As a community, we have developed a deeper understanding of compassion and its relationship with emerging technologies. The original Phoenix Project mandate sought to restore balance to human compassion, which we understood to be threatened by technologies. This threat is real and persistent; compassion requires vigilant study and protection. Certainly, technologies should not be celebrated uncritically as forces of positive change. However, as I argue in the opening chapter, we now recognize that technologies must not only be countered as opponents but also recruited as allies.

To create this book, we assembled an outstanding group of authors equipped to ponder various aspects of compassion through a lens of technology. We asked them, where possible, to find the middle road between unconvincing optimism and paralyzing cynicism. Although we gave authors no constraint of scope or focus, we asked them to embrace one assumption: the assumption that among industries currently buffeted by technological change, healthcare is uniquely anchored in human compassion. On this point we did not invite debate.

OVERVIEW

We did, however, give authors great latitude in conceiving of compassion and how to achieve it. While emergent technologies are the impetus for this book, compassion remains the primary focus. Each chapter examines an aspect of compassionate care. Working from varied points of view, the authors consider how compassion is currently practised, and they imagine a future in which compassion guides the way through a changing technological landscape.

The book is divided into two parts. The chapters in the first part are grouped together because each one reflects explicitly upon the meaning of compassion, urging us to think about the term in more nuanced or more critical ways. Wiljer, Strudwick, and Crawford use a prominent definition of compassion to think precisely about how technologies mediate compassionate care across changing digital health ecosystems. Rowland and Johannesen bring us back to first principles, asking what it means to recognize and respond to the suffering of others. Paton, Naidu, Richardson, Kumagai, and Kuper implore us to not limit compassionate acts to our own points of view or to the suffering of a privileged few. They ask us, instead, to expand our view from compassion to equity. These chapters all grapple with the meaning of compassion. They help us to be mindful in our efforts to advance compassionate care.

This emphasis upon cultivating compassion extends into the second part of the book. Here, the authors consider how compassion may be promoted, and how it may be threatened, by and for different individuals within healthcare organizations. Maunder, Chaukos, and Lawson consider the pressing problem of burnout among healthcare workers, attending to its underlying causes and corresponding strategies for showing care *toward* those who work daily to provide it. It is ironic and important that this chapter was written based on extensive research of the SARS experience. Though they could not have imagined COVID-19 when they set out to pen their chapter, they share wisdom that could not be more relevant today.

Mallette, Rose, and Spadoni grapple with the daunting challenge that educators face in preparing themselves and their students for an uncertain future as "curious, compassionate practitioners." Tassone,

Shaver, Lowe, Creede, and Parker offer a model of compassionate leadership that helps us to navigate changing contexts by keeping sight of our shared purpose and remaining attuned to our own and others' values, needs, and potential. Leaders include both the advocates of compassion who are distributed throughout organizations and those senior administrators who are charged with setting organizational priorities. Both have pivotal roles to play in creating and sustaining healthcare systems that are guided by a compassionate purpose. Martimianakis, Khan, Stergiopoulos, Briggs, and Fisman consider how organizations can support compassionate care in tangible ways by attending to structure, culture, and process, incorporating compassion into all levels of organizational planning.

Together, the authors in part two of this book suggest actions and principles that can be taken up by anyone – be it in a hospital, a hospice, or a home – to establish and inspire a culture of compassion.

Acknowledgments

This book is the result of the combined efforts of many people who dream of and work for a better, more compassionate healthcare system. Their aspirations and enthusiasm sustained this work.

The authors would like to recognize Sarah Whyte for her extraordinary dedication to this book, working intimately with all of the chapter authors and the editors to realize an integrated and compelling narrative.

We also thank the members of the AMS Phoenix community – fellows, researchers, partners, and advisers – who contributed to the thinking and knowledge explored in this text and who provided support and encouragement along the journey.

We are grateful to Kyla Madden and the team at McGill-Queen's University Press for support from the idea of the book through to its publication.

Anne Avery and Rachel Holden provide support every day to help AMS realize its goal of advancing compassionate care.

Finally, as sponsor for this work, the AMS Board – both current and past – has been a driving force to ask continuously how we can effectively inspire real change in health professions' education and practice. Their commitment to and unwavering support of the idea that compassionate care is the core to healthcare, and that technology can enable this, has propelled this work forward.

WITHOUT COMPASSION,
THERE IS NO HEALTHCARE

Technology, Compassion, and the Future of Healthcare

Brian D. Hodges

THE CHANGING LANDSCAPE OF HEALTH
PROFESSIONAL WORK

Emergent technologies will change the future of health professional work, rendering some tasks and professions obsolete.

Healthcare is strongly resistant to change. Despite the dramatic technological changes ahead, healthcare institutions and professions have been slow to prepare. Yet, as a teacher and chief medical officer in one of Canada's largest healthcare systems, I am regularly asked by students to help them understand what they will be doing in the future. In some cases, they have heard ominous predictions. Professor Geoffrey Hinton of Google and the University of Toronto has famously suggested, for example, that there will be no need for radiologists in ten years.

Simply reassuring the next generation of health professionals that they will continue to have a role is not enough. Students learning to be health professionals today need an education that will prepare them for a rapidly changing context. Much of what their teachers do today will not be what they themselves will do in the future. They must face this truth squarely, as must their teachers – a challenge taken up by Mallette and colleagues in chapter 5 of this book. Current health professionals are also confronting the challenge of practicing as experts while preparing themselves for very different workplaces.

Consider an example. At the Princess Margaret Cancer Centre in Toronto, a new AI-enabled treatment planning system was installed last year, initially for use with breast cancer patients requiring radiation therapy. Formerly, professionals caring for such patients would create a treatment plan to guide the machines that deliver powerful radiation. A treatment plan requires careful calculation of the dose, size, and strength of the radiation beam. Treatment must be located precisely on the patient's body. Incorrect calculations can lead to ineffective treatment or, in rare cases, radiation burns. For decades, a team of three professionals has created those plans: an oncologist, a radiation therapist, and a medical physicist. Together they analyze and integrate data from CT and MRI scans, other tests, and patients' charts. Until recently, the planning process averaged three to four hours per patient.

When I visited the Radiation Medicine Program or Radiation Oncology Department at Princess Margaret Cancer Centre recently, what I saw was amazing: using the new treatment planning system that once took three to four hours now takes about four minutes. Reducing a critical process in our hospital from hours to mere minutes is a tectonic shift in the work of the breast cancer radiation clinic. What happens to the time found through automation? Will that "gift of time" be reinvested into a better patient experience, into high quality and safety, or perhaps simply into the treatment of more patients? Among the hundreds of professionals at Princess Margaret Cancer Centre, there is great anticipation about the promise of emerging technologies such as this one but also a degree of apprehension (Gillan, Harnett, et al. 2018). What will be the future work of these professionals, and how will it change the experience of their patients?

It is sometimes (falsely) presumed that the changes wrought by technology will largely occur in tertiary hospital environments. Yet one of the most compelling examples I have recently encountered is an AI-driven system used in the community at the very front line of care. A simple smart phone or tablet equipped with an app allows community-based personal support workers, chiropodists, nurses, and family doctors to assess a diabetic foot wound. The pixilation of smart phone cameras is now sophisticated enough to analyze the micro-vascular structure (healthiness of the blood supply) of a wound and to determine whether care should be conservative (dressings, antibiotics, etc.) or rather urgent (hospital care) to prevent an amputation. Even in a hospital lab, this analysis for the prediction of healing has never been possible before. Phones and cameras have enabled the collection and interpretation of numerous data points. This is an amazing advance in terms of bringing care closer to patients. But it will also change which professionals do what and in what sequence to diagnose and treat diabetic foot ulcers.

The rhetoric of technological change can sometimes be overblown. Not all ominous predictions come to pass, and many that do will involve a slower evolution. In the 1980s, when I was a medical student, early electrocardiogram machines provided a rudimentary interpretation of a heart rhythm, but it was not a very reliable interpretation and it didn't displace the interpretation of a physician. Only recently have we developed more powerful computers with machine-learning capabilities that can spot cardiac anomalies just as well as humans can. Whatever the pace, however, professional scopes of practice are changing. The work of health professionals will be reconfigured substantially in coming years. Some functions, and perhaps some professions, may become obsolete even before the current generation retires.

We can predict with confidence that the work of health professionals will change. It is quite another matter to predict *how* it will change. Which roles will be enhanced, transformed, or replaced by machines? As sophisticated as technologies have become in conducting technical tasks, we intuitively believe that some things are so complex that only a human can achieve them. Could a computer ever detect and effectively respond to a patient's fear or sadness? Could it deliver bad news or weigh ethical options? Would we want it to? The next section explores some of these questions.

WHAT WILL WE NEED HUMANS FOR?

The changes to professional work will likely run deep, extending beyond routine tasks. They may disrupt the very foundations of the professions.

Predicting the future is an exercise fraught with risk. Yet science fiction sometimes provides the first accurate sketches. In 1983, a *Toronto Star* journalist asked the futurist writer Isaac Asimov to predict what the world would be like in 2019 (Johnson 2018). Many of his predictions have borne out. He wrote, for example, that computerization would "undoubtedly continue onward inevitably" and that the "mobile computerized object" would "penetrate the home." The increasing complexity of society, he predicted, would make it impossible to live without this technology. Computers would disrupt work habits and replace old jobs with ones that are radically different while robotics would kill "routine clerical and assembly-line jobs." Further, society would need a "vast change in the nature of education" such that "entire populations" would become computer-literate and able to deal with a high-tech world. Finally, and presciently, he noted that this transition would be rapid and difficult for many.

While Asimov was right in many ways, the pace of our adaptation to technological change in healthcare has been slower than he predicted. He imagined that we would have completed a major transition in our educational systems by 2019, and this has not occurred. He may have underestimated the kinds of jobs that would be affected by emerging technologies as well. Though there is no doubt that much "routine" work has already been replaced by automation, what is becoming apparent is that computerized systems will also impact more complex work such as medical diagnosis, a domain currently reserved for physicians.

In their book *The Future of the Professions* (2015), Oxford professors Richard Susskind and Daniel Susskind caution against the assumption that machines will take over only routine tasks and that human professionals will always be needed for work that is inherently complex. They note that the interpretation of digital images (e.g., X-rays, photographs, scans, or pathology slides) is indeed complex *for humans.* However, such tasks are rather straightforward for computers. A simple *routine* versus *complex* taxonomy is therefore not sufficient to predict what human health professionals will be needed for in the future.

In fact, no one will be unaffected by the coming technological transformations. As Asimov suggested, they may be "difficult for many." This makes it timely to ask: What will happen to the radiologists and radiology technologists, dermatologists and nurses, ophthalmologists and optometrists, oncologists and radiation therapists whose work is displaced, replaced, or transformed by technology?

This book imagines a future in which health professionals are no longer the sole owners of medical knowledge and dispensers of wisdom, nor the most adept or dexterous operators of precision instruments. A profound shift in what knowledge is and how medical procedures are performed is underway. That much is clear. But what about that most human of healthcare domains: compassion? Can we imagine that technology will ever play a meaningful role in listening empathically, understanding deeply, or offering comfort? The next section challenges a too-tempting dichotomy that humans are compassionate and technologies are not.

HUMANS AND TECHNOLOGIES AS ALLIES IN COMPASSIONATE CARE

In order to understand what kinds of work humans will be needed to do, we first need to acknowledge that humans and technologies are not opponents. Together, they create an urgent need for compassion – and only together are they likely to address that need.

So an AI-enabled computer can read an X-ray. But surely, people say to me, a computer cannot replace human compassion. If the emphasis is on the word *replace*, I ultimately share this conviction. Our case will be built on thin ground, however, if we assume that humans inherently demonstrate compassion and that technologies inherently threaten it. This book is devoted to exploring and championing the importance of compassion from every angle, including how technologies might be able to extend or amplify human compassion. That said, the editors and authors of this book are not uncritical champions of technology: the introduction of deep learning, AI, data analytics, and robots must also include a clear-eyed and critical look at how technology can work against compassionate care, and the book addresses that question too.

Neither are we naïve about the degree to which health professionals and institutions demonstrate compassion today. Though it is safe to assume that most health professionals have the *ability* to demonstrate compassion, professionals and patients will be the first to admit that in busy hospitals, clinics, and communities at large, compassion is often the first thing to evaporate in the push toward greater efficiency. Organizations may commonly cite compassionate care as a guiding value, but – as Martimianakis and colleagues argue in chapter 7 of this book – translating that value into practice requires tangible commitments across all levels of organizational planning. Far from finding consistent compassionate care, encounters with healthcare systems and the humans who run them may actually increase distress or even foster patients' suffering.

For this reason, we must be honest about the need to bolster the compassionate orientation of healthcare professionals and institutions in all forms. This has been an imperative, and a struggle, for hundreds of years. But as we enter the new technological era, we must begin to ask whether humans could actually collaborate with technologies such as computers and robots to advance compassionate care. While it is essential to understand the uniquely *human* dimensions of compassionate healthcare, it is also important to explore how technologies might be part of the solution.

In advocating for compassion in this book, therefore, we do not situate humans in opposition to technologies. Instead we ask, If compassion is essential in healthcare, *what deployment of human abilities and what technologies together will be most effective?* Each chapter of this book takes up a different dimension of the challenge. Across a variety of domains, the authors ask, What is compassion? How can humans ensure that healthcare remains compassionate in an era of emerging and disruptive technologies?

FLEXIBLE, ADAPTABLE HEALTHCARE PROFESSIONALS

The professions will survive only if they are versatile, focusing not only on knowledge and skills – which will undoubtedly change – but also on the overarching purpose of healthcare. Compassion and human connection are central to that purpose.

New technologies in workplaces of all kinds are challenging our notions about what core elements constitute any job or profession. Industries outside of healthcare provide compelling examples of transformation on a massive scale that resulted from automation more than a decade ago. Successful transformation relies on flexibility and adaptability of the workforce. For example, a recent summary of a report from the Royal Bank of Canada (2018, n.p.) argues that many jobs, even in what were thought to be disparate fields, are in fact connected by a similar set of foundational skills: "Musicians and paramedics might not seem to have a lot in common, but both jobs require high levels of focus, excellent analytical skills, and attention to detail. It takes upgrading only four skills for someone to transition from dental assistant to graphic designer."

While, of course, a great deal of specialized education differentiates a surgeon from a psychiatrist, this line of thinking is valuable to healthcare too. It directs our attention to foundational elements that underpin professional expertise rather than simply specific stores of knowledge or unique procedural skills. This line of thinking also opens the door to more flexible pathways to competence in the health professions than currently exist.

If a radiologist is no longer needed to read X-rays, is a radiologist no longer needed? Perhaps this is the wrong question. When a radiology resident asks me to speculate about their future, the challenge is to decode the foundational elements of their work that are likely to remain true, even if AI takes over some of the specific tasks that constitute the work today. Rather than thinking of radiologists as specialists who read X-rays, it is more useful to think of them as professionals who use various technologies to visualize the interior of the body for the purpose of medical diagnosis and treatment. This definition helps students and educators to focus on how technologies serve these specific functions and purposes. It also helps radiology residents to focus on learning about the technologies themselves – how they transform the human body into images and, critically, what biases and errors of interpretation they can introduce.

There is another consideration, and this one is crucial. Some of my radiologist colleagues tell me that the future of their profession lies in developing greater focus on the interface with other medical colleagues and with patients. I realized that I had held a stereotype of radiologists as doctors who sit in a dark room reading X-rays, until a colleague said, "I think the future of our profession lies in working closely with medical colleagues and patients to help them determine which technologies to use and how to make sense of the findings." He told me that he had started to work shifts in the emergency department to do just that. "We have to re-emphasize the human interaction part of our specialty."

The twentieth century involved a great deal of work by educators to define what it means to be a competent health professional in different roles. This work took the form of detailed (and often territorial) *competence frameworks* and *scopes of practice* documents. Such documents laid out all the knowledge and skills that students must learn to pass high stakes professional examinations. These frameworks have often been undergirded by Miller's Pyramid, a hierarchical model that articulates competence at four levels: knows, knows how, shows, and does. From this framework an enormous system of assessment and certification has grown, involving professional colleges, accreditation bodies, and certification procedures. It is now almost impossible to pivot from one area of professional expertise to another without enduring a long program of retraining and recertification. And it is becoming clear that this edifice of health professions education, certification, and accreditation is not suited to the future of health-care; it does not foster the flexibility and adaptability that the future healthcare workforce will need.

The changing landscape of practice also makes evident that specific domains of sub-specialized knowledge and skills are not enough. Health professionals master a lot of knowledge, including both the memorization of facts and the application of information in practice, such as diagnosis. They also master a bevy of technical skills, ranging from the simple taking of blood pressure to the most complex of surgical procedures. Yet for all that knowledge and skill, the practice of health professionals, regardless of specialty or profession, is held together by a remarkably similar core purpose: to care for other humans in ways that alleviate suffering. That is healthcare's compassionate purpose. It is therefore alarming to note that some competence frameworks have lost sight of compassion altogether. Research supported by AMS Healthcare in the last decade has shown an almost complete disappearance of the word *compassion* (and, more astoundingly still, the word *care*) from the competence frameworks in medicine and nursing (Whitehead, Kuper, et al. 2014).

While specialized knowledge and skill will always have great importance, as computers develop abilities that rival human brains, the interpersonal domain may become our greatest differentiator. From a strictly economic perspective, "competencies that are complementary to machine prediction will become more valuable in the future, while competencies that are substitutes for machine prediction will become less valuable" (Li, Kulasegaram, and Hodges 2019, 623). In many ways this is a positive realization; it recognizes that our human capacity for compassion is much less specialty specific than is our cognitive knowledge – and that without it healthcare cannot exist. Put another way, all the knowledge held in internet clouds combined with the most sophisticated pattern recognition of AI, bolstered by the dexterity of the latest robots will not be sufficient to create high-quality healthcare. These technological capabilities, extraordinary as they are, must be combined with the human capacity for compassion in order to deliver the complete healthcare package.

But in order for healthcare professionals, educators, and patients to fully understand how human compassion will fit into healthcare systems of the future, we first need to take a closer look at what is happening to the domains of professional knowledge and skills that advanced technologies are disrupting. We must consider what health professionals may no longer be doing.

KNOWLEDGE IS IN THE CLOUDS

Well-established factual knowledge, once central to professional expertise, is readily replaced by computers.

The television show *Star Trek: Voyager* gave us the first glimpse of a holographic doctor. In creating the character of "The Doctor," the writers anticipated what an AI-enabled computer diagnostic system might be like. Though a real actor played The Doctor, it strikes no one as odd today that the knowledge necessary for the practice of medicine could be stored in a non-human database activated by voice. In fact, most of us already use this technology every day in our phones. You can ask a smartphone, "What is a normal level of blood potassium?" or "Does penicillin interact with grapefruit juice?" and expect to get a meaningful answer. For this reason, there is little justification for health professional students to memorize thousands of pages of biochemical formulae, anatomical parts, or drug names and interactions. Memorization has become, in the view of many, a waste of cognitive resources. Most of medicine's factual knowledge is not held in human brains; it is accessed from computer databases.

Databases of factual knowledge also enable patients to be more participatory in their own care. Many people, with and without professional training, consult the internet to learn about medical problems. As a physician, I regularly use the internet to find evidence related to the treatment of my patients, but I also use it in relation to my own health. Recently, I found a video that helped me to treat my sprained ankle. (It has been a long time since I completed my generalist training!) Patients and families can access the same information as health professionals. Imagine that you develop repetitive strain injury. Are you likely to go through the trouble of getting an appointment with a healthcare professional if you can easily access and understand information provided online? I recently had just that experience and found an excellent video of exercises to counteract the repetitive pain I get from too much typing.

Such well-established factual and procedural knowledge – similar to what the ancient philosopher Aristotle termed *episteme* – has traditionally informed the central dimensions of professional expertise. In the foreseeable future, a role will persist for specialized knowledge and for the interpretation of complex signs and symptoms. This role, however, will continue to diminish. Increasingly, databases can be accessed for the purposes of analysis and learning directly by computers, such that computers can master more extensive and complex forms of knowledge. They are also able to provide informative probabilistic analyses of diagnostic signs and symptoms. Machine learning and AI will continue to evolve rapidly and will be widely used to support human interpretations and judgments of patterns of illness and disease. Sometimes, people will bypass health professionals and go directly to the internet for interpretation of symptoms or recommendations for treatment.

This suggests an emerging role for human health professionals. Much information on the internet is of poor quality, and there will be a role for professionals to help patients deal with the clouds of facts, many of which are replete with biases. Even those facts that are effectively uncontested need to be appropriately selected and applied. Human professionals will be needed to help people navigate, evaluate, and interpret competing perspectives and available options. Eric Topol, author of a landmark report to England's National Healthcare Service, observes, "The new medicine envisioned will require extensive education and training of the clinician workforce and the public, with cultivation of a cross-disciplinary approach that includes data scientists, computer scientists, engineers, [and] bio-informaticians, in addition to the traditional mix of pharmacists, nurses and doctors" (Topol 2019b, 6).

Perhaps the first task for this large and diversified healthcare team is to understand much more about the differences between humans and computers in how they think and what kinds of errors they're prone to make. Only then will we know how humans and machines can work most effectively together.

RECOGNIZING PATTERNS: SKIN LESIONS, CHIHUAHUAS, AND BLUEBERRY MUFFINS

Computers and human experts each excel at pattern recognition in different ways – and each is vulnerable to different kinds of errors. Humans are ultimately responsible for understanding the specific power and limits of technologies, and for deploying them appropriately.

Humans have highly developed abilities to take in thousands of pieces of diverse sensory information and rapidly form an impression. Health professionals learn to do this quickly from seeing hundreds of patients, and they test their initial impressions by asking careful confirmatory questions and analyzing physical signs and laboratory results. Consequently, health professionals become experts at recognizing patterns.

Computers are also very good at pattern recognition. Computer-based pattern recognition involves digital algorithms programmed by humans. Increasingly, in the case of machine learning, computers themselves will also be able to generate and modify algorithms as they interact with large data sets. Hundreds of such algorithms already operate behind the scenes in our daily lives.

Algorithms are nothing new. They have existed as long as there have been computers and were used by humans long before that. A decision tree that helps a doctor assemble signs and symptoms into a diagnosis is a simple algorithm. What has changed is the sophistication of algorithms and the speed at which they can be automated and employed. Whereas algorithms were once of interest only to computer programmers, today they govern our daily lives. When we interact with the internet, algorithms make analytic judgments *about us*, by comparing our personal qualities or features against a database. For example, search engines such as Google use algorithms to determine what advertisements to make visible to us. An algorithm incorporates data about everything we have done and shared online: past searches, purchases, personal demographic data (often harvested from social media), where we live and shop, our age, gender, and culture. It then makes predictions about what we will be interested in, what we are likely to click on, and what we might purchase. The algorithms are used to push customized information to us.

This is also how algorithms work in healthcare. Many pieces of information about you – including your medical history, CT and MRI scans, X-rays, blood samples, biopsies, and psychological tests – can be compared to a huge database of other people's information. By comparing your data to norms, computers predict the presence or absence of diseases and probabilities of future events

Yet pattern recognition is neither completely objective nor neutral. Both humans and machines can make errors, though they tend to do so in different ways. Take, for example, a popular meme that illustrates the challenge for AI of distinguishing a chihuahua's face from a blueberry muffin. If the two little eyes and nose are similar in configuration to three blueberries on a muffin top, a computer can confuse the images. This example is perhaps something of an urban legend now; AI can generally (though imperfectly) pass this test. The nature of this error nevertheless illustrates an important point: a five-year-old human child would not confuse a dog and a muffin.

An interesting question, as healthcare moves forward with machine-human collaboration, is whether computer-generated predictions will be able to support patients in ways that are qualitatively similar to the guidance of human health professionals, or whether they will simply mimic that support in a superficial fashion. Will Dr Google's advice be simply watered-down medical care or could it contribute a valuable new dimension? One area of potential added value is prognostication. Humans can easily miss subtle patterns in layers of complex patient data. A study aiming to predict survival in patients with heart failure, for example, showed that an AI-enabled computer was better able than physicians to integrate the data from scans and tests with eight years of chart data, resulting in more accurate predictions of survival by the computer than by the physicians. This is perhaps unsurprising, given the cognitive difficulty for a human of amassing and integrating so much information. No physician has time to thoroughly read eight years of charts.

So humans and computers each have strengths, weaknesses, and blinds spots in performing pattern recognition. What is critical is that we understand (and teach) the specific biases and types of errors to which human and computer processes are prone. These biases and errors may be radically different. To avoid them, health professionals in the future will need to have a much better understanding of how human and artificial minds work, and how they work together. It will not be sufficient in healthcare to use information technologies in the way that we tend to use search engines like Google – entering questions into a blank box, which uses a process that we don't understand, and simply accepting the answer as correct.

But it is also fallacy to believe that human judgment is free of bias. Many studies confirm that humans are prone to all sorts of distortions in recognizing patterns and making judgments. Some derive from transient human weaknesses like fatigue or distraction. Others derive from ingrained cognitive biases, such as the halo effect of interpreting new information through old assumptions, or the recency effect of being influenced by the case seen just before a new one. Still others derive from pervasive social biases, such as the stereotyping of racial, linguistic, gender, and cultural factors. Human judgment is replete with bias. What is becoming visible is a new concern that when humans build computers, we may create algorithms that actually amplify human biases.

In her book *Algorithms of Oppression*, Safiya Umoja Noble (2018) illustrates this problem with a simple example. She shows the very different information that was returned from searches of the internet with the terms "Black girls" versus "white girls." The former search returned a high number of pornographic and racist sites, while the latter produced such things as preppy college websites and beauty products. These differences could be explained because the algorithms that determined associated terms were derived from other past searches. In other words, the search algorithms built on and amplified very human, and in this case racist, biases. Similar research in the social sciences reveals that algorithms can embed discrimination when they are used to determine who is eligible for social programs such as housing or employment benefits (Eubanks 2018). In chapter 3 of this book, Paton and colleagues build on examples such as these to show how compassion is interconnected with the broader concept of equity.

This points to an important role for human professionals who wish to use new technologies that provide diagnoses and prognoses in a way that is compassionate. Far from assuming that computer-based systems will be more objective, human health professionals will likely have to be even more vigilant in ensuring that diagnostic systems are fair, accurate, and objective.

WISDOM GOES BEYOND PATTERN RECOGNITION

Computerized algorithms can be insensitive to cultural and situational specificities. Humans should strive not only for practical knowledge, which involves recognizing and applying patterns but also for wisdom: judgment in specific situations that integrates factual and technical knowledge with ethical and interpersonal sensitivity.

When a doctor or nurse interacts with an algorithm-driven system to determine if a patient's test results are normal or to predict their clinical outcome, it will matter if they also know what data were used to create the database, what the algorithms are looking for, and what sorts of erroneous assumptions or errors might be made.

Such issues are pressing today because healthcare applications using AI are already coming online. The Food and Drug Administration in the United States has recently licensed for clinical use an AI-driven diagnostic system that can classify skin lesions (FDA 2019). It is easy to take a picture of a new brown spot on your arm and ask the system the likelihood that it is a freckle, a benign mole, or a cancerous melanoma. The system is accurate and will be a boon to both patients and health professionals, particularly given how hard it is to access a dermatologist. To perform this remarkable task, the system had to be trained. Training involved teaching the AI system to recognize skin lesions by showing it pictures and telling it the right answer. The system became quite reliable after it had seen nearly 130,000 images together with the correct diagnosis (Esteva, Kuprel, et al. 2017). The AI system learned to rapidly and accurately identify skin lesions it has never seen before and to triage patients into high-risk or low-risk groups for follow-up. But what is the risk of such applications? The pictures used to train such systems primarily represent Caucasian patients. How will such systems perform when classifying skin lesions from people with other skin tones (Lashbrook 2018)?

At a higher level of complexity than skin lesions, AI systems are available to recognize human emotions and behaviours. Some of the inventors would have us believe that computers even have the power to "eliminate human bias" in interpreting patterns of human behaviour. Brown (2107) describes how emotion recognition technologies detect "subtle 'micro-expressions' associated with joy, trust, fear, surprise, sadness, disgust, and anger" in order to quickly and accurately predict people's emotions and motivations. Such descriptions beg careful consideration of how those characteristics were defined and compared to what set of "normal" data. These limits and biases often remain hidden from view. We surely cannot call this technology accurate or indeed compassionate if we believe, as I do, that compassion requires authentic understanding.

A skin lesion, serum potassium measurement, or picture of a retina presents specific questions and concrete data for computer analysis. By contrast, most visits to a health professional are initiated by more ambiguous patient complaints or problems. Unlike reading an image, understanding a complaint (or set of symptoms) is more involved than simple visual pattern recognition because it requires attention to physical, physiological, biochemical, social, and psychological elements all at once. This integrated understanding is a key element in compassionate care. If a clinician is to generate understanding with a goal of relieving suffering then they must employ careful observation and skilled inquiry to interpret multi-dimensional data. That data may also include what is not said at all. Consider a woman who complains of abdominal pain and has subtle abrasions on her arm – symptoms that make little sense until the physician or nurse recognizes that she averts her eyes, a clue to ask about domestic violence.

Even health professionals who are skilled in the use of newer technologies voice caution about their application in healthcare. Dr Isaac Kohane, Chair of Harvard Medical School's Department of Biomedical Informatics, is skilled in the application of "big data." Yet in an article titled "The Beauty of 'Small Data' in Medicine" (2018), he shares a cautionary tale from his training. Kohane recounts how he met a nine-year-old boy referred to his clinic for short stature. His first impression was that the child didn't seem very short, though a family photo showed that the child was shorter than his seven-year-old brother. Normal practice would have been to plot the boy's growth, perhaps order an X-ray and blood tests, and send his family home with reassurance. But Kohane's teacher, a man with great experience in child development, noticed a subtle abnormality on the growth chart of the child that prompted him to repeat the measurements and recommend a brain scan. The scan revealed a benign brain tumour that was (happily) removed by a neurosurgical team. Dr Kohane's message? The case "marked the beginning of a long education on the value of small data – that is, the clinical impact of a small number of reliable measurements on a single patient." He notes that his own role as a "big data practitioner" offers all the more reason "to remember how much can be done with careful, meticulous consideration of data coming from a single patient" (Kohane 2018, n.p.)

Compassion requires such close attention to the symptoms and experiences of each individual. It goes well beyond the simple application of an established database to recognize a pattern. Integrating signs and symptoms with clinical experience, practical wisdom, and an ethical framework is far more complex. Compassion is not only specific to individuals but also to cultures. Eliminating biases might be highly desirable from the point of view of reducing superficial diagnostic assumptions and errors; however, what does bias mean in sophisticated, culturally determined human behaviours and emotions? Consider eye contact. Many standardized checklists of communication skills start with the item "makes eye contact" at the top. Such checklists constitute simple algorithms for judging trustworthiness. Humans attach significant meaning to the act of making or avoiding eye contact. If someone averts their eyes, others often suspect that they are hiding something. This interpretation is built into algorithms used at airports to detect suspicious travellers. How long until a computer-assisted diagnostic system includes eye contact within assessments of depression, anxiety, or perhaps even truthfulness concerning personal relations or drug use?

Yet, in Indigenous cultures, making eye contact is considered rude. I have worked with Indigenous peoples in Canada's Arctic communities who tell me that direct eye contact with a stranger feels like inappropriate touching. For some Indigenous peoples, and indeed in many cultures, avoiding eye contact is a sign of respect. If this interpretation of eye averting is not captured in an automated system (perhaps because few Indigenous people were part of the database), the system would have a built-in bias that could lead to significant problems of interpretation and of understanding.

Because compassion is in part about understanding, any technology that we imagine to have compassionate uses must be evaluated through a socio-cultural lens. When health professionals use machines to aid in diagnosing a skin lesion or assessing mental capacities and behaviours, they must be vigilant about what algorithms include, what they leave out, and to what databases and norms they are compared. Further, as algorithms begin to help control who can and cannot access healthcare and social services, very human biases related to gender, race, religion, and other socio-demographics may too easily be built in. Ultimately, it must be humans who maintain vigilance to ensure ethical and compassionate uses of technology.

WHEN COMPUTERS LEARN THE MEDICAL GAZE[1]

Technologies have introduced distance between healthcare providers and patients. This distance has often been a threat to compassion. Health professionals need to be aware of this distance and find new ways to foster presence.

All medical students are shown the picture in figure 0.1. It is in some ways the primal image of medical care. A caring doctor gazes at a poor, sick child, while a mother weeps and a stoic father looks on with concern. There are some stereotypes at play here, but in essence,

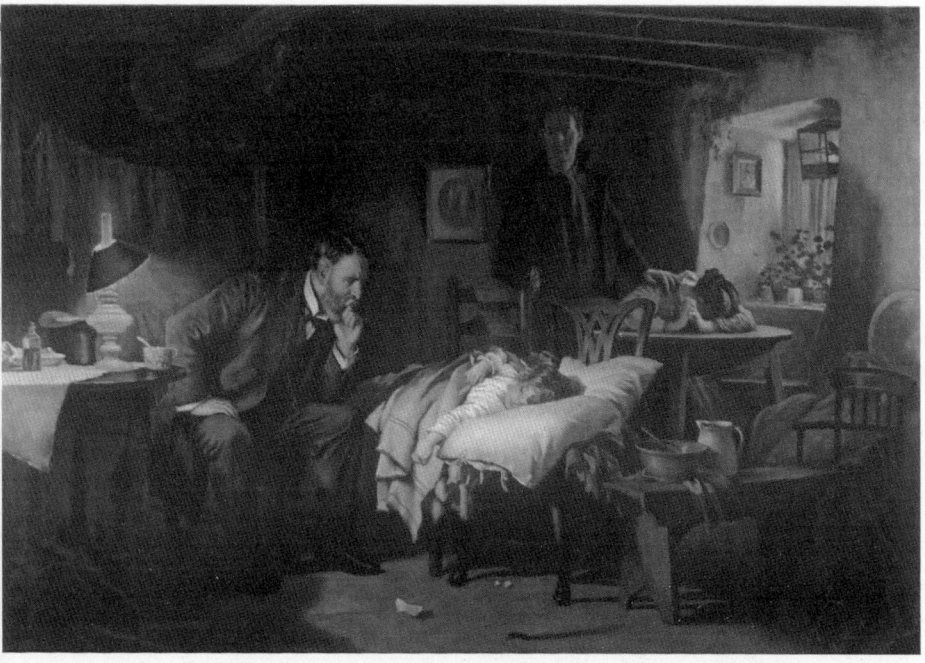

Figure 0.1 *The Doctor* by Luke Fildes (1891) illustrates the medical gaze

this is how many continue to imagine that a healthcare professional brings compassion to patients. Philosopher Michel Foucault, in his book *The Birth of the Clinic*, describes this *gaze* as a knowing and penetrating way of looking at a patient. *The Birth of the Clinic* traces the origin of the concept of clinical medicine itself. Though written a half century ago, it continues to serve as a relevant history of the ideas that underpin healthcare. Prior to the eighteenth century, the practice of medicine was largely mystical: theories abounded of misplaced organs, blocked humours, wind in the joints, and flows of energy. The rise of scientific medicine, with its dissections, experiments, and animal studies changed all that.

But Foucault notes another change in this seminal work. He cautions that this gaze – the objectifying, apparently neutral, scientific, medical gaze – could, in fact, turn patients into objects of study, rather like the way one looks down a microscope at an insect. Today, his work helps to explain how health professionals sometimes drift from caring for patients to studying them as objects. Sometimes, in our best attempts to help people, we stop seeing the people and begin to focus more on the diseases, the cells, or the X-rays that come from them.

The danger of objectification began long before the rise of AI and robots, but the objectifying medical gaze becomes more powerful still when a machine does the gazing. While a human health professional may be prone to inattentiveness, we can return to awareness of our patients' humanity. There is no such awareness for an automated system. Human health professionals must ensure that patients' experiences are recognized and acknowledged – that their treatment is *humane*, as they interact with increasingly non-human technologies.

Some technologies will develop superficial forms of empathy. Some might even seem polite or convincing. Indeed, all machines should be designed with caring as one goal of the experience for people who use them. In chapter 1 of this book, Wiljer and colleagues begin the important work of mapping how technologies can mediate compassionate care in a variety of ways across healthcare ecosystems. Nevertheless, human presence will never be entirely replaceable: a machine alone can never have a compassionate aim. One main function of human healthcare professionals in the future may be to recognize the power that simply being present has to reduce the objectification of patients. Judith John is a long-time patient activist at Toronto's University Health Network. She advises new health professional students and seasoned veterans alike: "I want you to be present for me" (John 2016).

The etymological root of the word *compassion* is "suffering with," which suggests that compassion requires human *presence* – a principle central to the discussion of patient engagement in chapter 2 of this book (by Rowland and Johannesen) and of compassionate leadership in chapter 6 (by Tassone and colleagues). If we value presence, it becomes problematic when technologies distract, displace, or diminish humans in their connections with each other. A simple example is the rise of people walking around the streets with their eyes fixed on their mobile phones. This common behaviour, reinforced by a perceived need for (or addiction to) *virtual* interaction, clearly interrupts human interaction in the physical world. Similarly, when a clinician turns her back on a patient to enter data into a computer, the human connection is partly broken. Leaving aside for the moment the possibility of technologies that can reinforce human interaction, it seems self-evident that patients will want to be known, cared for, and comforted by other humans – to feel their presence and to benefit from their attentiveness, at least sometimes in the course of their care. It also seems self-evident that many, if not most, who work in healthcare are governed by the value they place on human interaction. Indeed, my personal suspicion is that the current epidemic of burnout among health professionals is largely driven by the diminution of human contact in our work environments. In chapter 4 of this book, Maunder and colleagues delve into supporting evidence: relationships are integral to fostering resilience and protecting against burnout. Healthcare work will face a mounting crisis if there is continued erosion of human presence and human interaction.

THE DISTANCE BETWEEN US

Amazing new technologies enhance clinical care, but they are often interposed in the physical space between health professional and patient. This can interfere with the human connection.

The *laying on of hands* has traditionally strengthened the relationship between patients and health professionals by creating a physical bond. There was a time when the physical examination was the core of medical diagnosis. When I trained in medical school thirty years ago, we learned about things such as "whispering pectoriloquy" (the sound of the whispered voice heard through a stethoscope) and diaphragmatic excursion (the movement of the diaphragm measured by tapping, or "percussing," with one's finger along the chest wall). Today, my students say, "Why would we do that? Don't we just get an X-ray or a 2-D echo?" Something has been lost, I think, in adopting these admittedly more accurate diagnostic tools. The physical exam was not about the diagnostic process alone. The physical contact also established human connection.

About two centuries ago, a physician in France named René T.H. Laënnec invented the stethoscope. Indeed, the stethoscope is a marvellous tool. From the first one – which was just a rolled up paper tube placed against the patient's chest – our diagnostic capability has been dramatically improved. With a stethoscope, a physician, nurse, or respiratory therapist can hear breath sounds, heart sounds, and bowel sounds with ease. A little later, a modification allowed physicians and midwives to hear the rapidly beating heart of a developing baby in a woman's abdomen.

The stethoscope, though, created a little physical space between the physician, nurse, or midwife and the people they examine. That small space has been growing wider and wider. Today the stethoscope is largely a historical object. Though many health professionals still carry one, it functions more as a symbol of a professional role rather than a tool in actual use (Bernstein 2016). Of course it still functions, just as it always did, but most of us now are thinking more about the human relationship when we use one.

I am mindful of when and how I touch my patients. As a medical psychiatrist in a large hospital, I work in intensive care units, on organ transplantation services, and in the emergency department. The patients I see are often confused or delirious. Some come to hospital with a psychiatric disorder such as depression or anxiety. It is really very difficult for anyone to be in a place like an intensive care unit. The lights are never turned off; the machines, such as respirators and intravenous pumps, whir and beep constantly. The healthcare professionals circulate on rounds at all hours of day and night. If I stand at the bedside in a starched white coat wearing a mask and only use my voice to communicate with a patient attached to all those machines, we are both cut off from the human relationship we need to have. So, I always place my hand on a patient's shoulder, hold their hand, or cradle their wrist, perhaps going through the motions of checking a pulse to normalize the touching. Thus a human connection is established.

When my own appendix ruptured in 2010, I was amazed to experience as a patient how little human contact there was when the diagnosis was made and communicated. My doctor reported to me, "The CT scan showed that you have a perforated appendix." I thought, Wow, the *CT scanner* made my diagnosis? Of course it was a human radiologist who examined the CT image, made a diagnostic conclusion, and called the emergency physician. But I never met the radiologist, and the emergency physician performed only a cursory examination of my abdomen. I had no actual connection with either.

Technologies can help with diagnosis and treatment, but they can also create new distances and barriers to human presence. This is particularly true of the most technologically intensive areas of care, such as surgery. Health professionals of the future working in these environments will need to find strategies, old and new, to forge human connections across increasing distances.

AUTOMATION AND TECHNICAL SKILLS

Technologies greatly extend the technical precision of humans. In surgery, these technical capacities are still deployed by human judgment – and patients tend to place their trust in humans.

While the cognitive domains of healthcare, including pattern recognition, diagnosis, and prognosis are undergoing transformation, there is an equally profound shift underway in technical skills. Consider how technology is changing brain surgery. At Toronto Western Hospital patients now commonly arrive in the morning, have a craniotomy (the skull opened or small holes created), then wires or shunts implanted or a tumour removed, all in time for them to return home the same evening.

How is it possible that performing a brain implant or removing a tumour has become same-day surgery? Many technologies have contributed to transforming what were once long, dangerous operations with many days in hospital into one-day procedures. Among them are improved surgical instruments, better sterilization, high-quality imaging, precision lenses for neurosurgeons, and anesthesia that removes all feeling of pain but allows patients to remain awake. Indeed, the success of all forms of surgery has dramatically improved in the last century. Today, aided by tiny rods and cameras, surgeons can operate in minute spaces where clumsy hands would do damage. These technologies are arguably compassionate because they improve outcomes while vastly decreasing the suffering of patients.

Even more dramatic is the arrival of surgical robots; they are extraordinary to watch. Though some robots look humanoid, with arms, legs, and heads, surgical robots are not like that. In fact, most robots do not look like humans. While mimicking human anatomy may have some advantages, we humans are actually rather limited in a number of ways. Human hands, while amazingly dexterous, for their size they do not work efficiently in small body cavities. Enter the surgical robot.

The first time I watched a surgical robot in action was in a gynecological operating room at Toronto General Hospital. While I had spent many weeks in surgery as a medical student and during my generalist training, it had been years since I had visited an operating room. I was immediately struck by the transformation. A woman (the patient) was suspended, anesthetized, from the ceiling by a series of straps and harnesses. One doctor (the anesthesiologist) sat near her overseeing the tubes delivering the sedation. Another doctor (the surgical assistant) stood by, observing as the metal rods of the robot moved in and out of tiny holes in the patient's abdomen. The surgeon herself was seated at a console across the room, facing a screen on which she could see inside the patient while she operated hand and foot controls. This is not the operating room of my training or that most people imagine.

Humans collaborating with machines such as surgical robots are changing what it means to work as a health professional. Robots are fast becoming our *team members*. Healthcare will require humans to do things, but increasingly machines are augmenting our steadiness, precision, reach, and accuracy. In the examples I have described, robotic systems take up some of the direct, technical work while humans use their judgment to deploy and monitor those systems. The impact on outcomes, such as healing and recovery time, is tremendous and positive. However, in the process, a new risk presents itself: the physical distance grows between professionals and the people they treat as technologies become intermediaries between clinician and patient.

Author of *The Digital Doctor* Robert Wachter remarks that healthcare's path to computerization "has been strewn with land mines, large and small. Medicine, our most intimately human profession, is being dehumanized by the entry of the computer into the exam room." He adds, "While someday the computerization of medicine will surely be that long-awaited 'disruptive innovation,' today it's often just plain disruptive: of the doctor-patient relationship, of clinicians' professional interactions and workflow, and of the way we measure and try to improve things" (Wachter 2015, xi).

In addition to the effects of growing physical distance, there is another consideration when machines join the healthcare team: they can fail. Who hasn't had the experience of a program crashing, or a computer rebooting to update software, at a critical moment? Such failures can cause human emotions to flare in machine-human encounters. But the stakes are even higher when machine failure arises in healthcare settings that are already characterized by emotional tension. What happens when a surgical robot reboots or a radiation therapy machine responds unpredictably or fails outright? A burgeoning literature documents the rising problem of failing medical devices (Ferrarese, Pozzi, et al. 2016; Hengstler, Enkel, and Duelli 2016). The radiation treatment team at the Princess Margaret is very aware of an infamous and devastating radiation machine failure that led to several deaths in the 1980s. As Jamie Lynch (2017, n.p.) remarks in a blog post titled "The Worst Computer Bugs in History," while such cases are extreme and rare, "they are worth studying for the insights they can offer into software development and deployment. These computer bugs left a significant impact on the people who experienced them, and we hope they'll offer valuable lessons we can all apply to our own work and projects."

A key issue in the evolution of human-machine technical skills, then, is learning to grapple with very human responses – the "significant impact on the people who experience them." An emerging phenomenon is called *computer rage* or *tech rage*, "an overwhelming emotion caused by frustration with one or more technological devices" (Shaw 2015). Neither computers nor robots are autonomously motivated by a sense of urgency. Nor do they feel fear or panic. Thus it falls to the humans who acquire, maintain, and operate machines to recognize and modulate their own emotions *and* those of the patients they are caring for when problems with technology arise.

Unfortunately, the challenge of dealing with the stressors of human-machine interaction and the problem of interpersonal distance between health professionals can converge. Consider a homecare nurse who cares for patients in the community and uses a telehealth system, a radiologist who works in her office in one country and interprets a CT scan taken in another country, or a gastroenterologist in a hospital who uses a machine-guided system to perform a biopsy. All of these professionals benefit from significant gains in automation and autonomy and from distributed models of care. But all of them work in ways that are more isolated and further removed from the colleagues with whom they can confer. A surgical fellow, shaken, recently told me that he experienced three different pieces of equipment failing during a critical operation. Though surgical fellows are fully qualified physicians, they are learning a subspecialty and still require support and supervision from experienced experts. In this case, a number of operating rooms were running simultaneously and the fellow was unable to reach his supervisor. Marshalling his creativity, with input from the nurses and anaesthetists, he managed to stop a serious hemorrhage. But he told me afterwards that it was all he could do to control his rage at the malfunctioning equipment. This fellow recognized that his emotions were significantly impinging on his problem-solving in the operation room. As he told me darkly, "Of course I can get someone by email or text, but that doesn't help any of us when all hell is breaking loose."

VIRTUAL EMPATHY AND COMPASSION?

Humans have a strong need for close emotional and physical contact. Mediated and virtual connectivity may impoverish human connections, becoming harmful when clinicians and patients need emotional support.

Research among our primate cousins shows that isolated individuals will die from a starvation for contact, and loneliness among humans is associated with increased mortality (Holt-Lunstad, Smith, et al. 2015). Many of today's new technologies, including the varied forms of social media, bring the promise of greater connectivity. Indeed, communication channels such as email, text, or social media can bridge distances and help form new connections. In healthcare, the rise of the "virtual" visit conducted over email or videoconference can augment accessibility to care. But we need to be careful with these technologies and not assume that they automatically confer the same value for human contact.

I saw a young man in my office recently for symptoms of depression. When I asked about his relationships, he told me that he had 107 friends. Of course, those were friends on social media. When I asked him how many people in his life he could trust, talk with face to face, and discuss his feelings with, the answer was zero. I learned that he had great difficultly talking casually with people at school or at the gym, and he found he was only able to communicate through the mediation of his mobile phone. I spent weeks helping him, little by little, learn the basics of sharing casual conversation with strangers and eventually meeting some new people "live." This is not to say that everyone suffers from interpersonal challenges as serious as this young man's, but there is a general trend to relate to one another via communication technologies, and the consequences of that trend warrant careful consideration.

As a physician, I provide support to my patients by email or text. Many of them find this comforting. However, I am aware of some early research revealing the limits of mediated communication in my own field. When our Department of Psychiatry at the University of Toronto began video consultations to the northern parts of Canada three decades ago, it quickly became clear that appointments via video conference were much more effective if the clinician and patient had already formed a personal, face-to-face relationship.

In some cases, patients may prefer virtual alternatives to traditional forms of communication. Talking with a human to book a clinic appointment, for instance, may be less desirable than having a good app that allows easy appointment reservations and automatic confirmation. Using a robust online system to access preoperative information may be preferable to driving across town, or farther, to hear it from a person at the hospital. On the one hand, many people already benefit from and appreciate the ability to see their laboratory results online in patient portals. On the other hand, non-human systems for such things as counselling, psychotherapy, or the delivery of bad news – all of which are being developed – may garner mixed feelings and results for patients. Among health professionals themselves, email and text are not the most supportive mediums for communicating in a crisis situation.

As we parse the value of different technologies in their ability to augment or detract from human presence, a nutritional analogy comes to mind. Diet soda looks and tastes much like food, but it's an illusion. There is no nutritional value in diet soda. It seems to me that many forms of communication in healthcare today provide a diet soda version of compassion: they appear to foster human relationships, but the value of the resulting connection is more illusory than real. Not all live human interactions are rich in compassion, of course. But the risk grows for meaningless communication and *pseudo-empathy* as the medium becomes more depersonalized. Most of us have experienced the phenomenon of receiving (or sending) an email message that we would never consider appropriate in face-to-face communication. Technological mediation of communication, and ultimately its connection to empathy and compassion, is complex. Mediated communication is not necessarily bad, but it does require good design. In healthcare, it is essential to understand how to build and sustain relationships that foster empathy, understanding, and ultimately compassion, regardless of the medium.

To function effectively, to support each other, to stay calm when there are problems, and to provide care that is compassionate, healthcare professionals need to be savvier at using mediated forms of communication with patients and with each other. Attention will have to be paid to limiting formats that compromise understanding or diminish empathy. Importantly, health professionals must pay attention to the effects of different technologies on their own well-being.

Dr Atul Gawande is a gifted medical writer and self-confessed technophile. Yet he draws strong links between the uptake of computerized processes and the burnout of health professionals: "Something's gone terribly wrong." He remarks, "Doctors are among the most technology-avid people in society; computerization has simplified tasks in many industries. Yet somehow we've reached a point where people in the medical profession actively, viscerally, volubly hate their computers" (Gawande 2018b, n.p.). While he holds a clear-eyed view that the tools available today greatly enhance our ability to collect, store, and analyze information, leading to better and safer diagnoses and treatments, he notes that much can be lost along the way. "The story of modern medicine is the story of our human struggle with complexity. Technology will, without question, continually increase our ability to make diagnoses, to peer more deeply inside the body and the brain, to offer more treatments. It will help us document it all – but not necessarily to make sense of it all. Technology inevitably produces more noise and new uncertainties" (Gawande 2018b, n.p.).

REDOUBLING THE COMMITMENT TO COMPASSION IN HEALTHCARE

Compassion has always been an anchor of healthcare. The technological revolution before us is a burning platform to restate and reinvigorate the commitment to compassionate healthcare.

As we have seen, all the knowledge and skill in the world are not sufficient to qualify as a good doctor or nurse. One needs years of experience to know when and how to deploy knowledge and skills in ways that enable compassionate care. This is true whether the knowledge is held in a computer database or the skills involve a robot. There are many elements of practical wisdom including judgment, reflection, and adaptation to context. And there is no quality more central to good healthcare than compassion. Myriad studies demonstrate that human relationships affect health outcomes: communication, empathy, and ultimately compassionate healthcare are all related to better treatment adherence, reduced anxiety, increased trust, less need for pain medication, and even better rates of recovery and survival.

It is time to take a hard look at how humans can work together with technologies to enhance these outcomes even further. But as the many examples I have discussed illustrate, this "working together" is not as straightforward as acquiring and installing a new computer or robot.

Consider one last example. Perhaps you saw the movie *Her*? Actress Scarlett Johansson plays the role of the computer operating system that speaks to the main character, Theodore, played by Joaquin Phoenix. When the film opens, Theodore has had a rough time: he is isolated, unhappy in his job, and has lost his partner. The computer operating system asks, "How are you feeling today?" and suggests, "I notice you didn't go to the gym this morning. Maybe you'd like me to arrange for you to go for dinner." We're not so very far from this today. The ability of AI to ask probing questions and to respond is rapidly advancing.

Do you think of this as compassion? Did the creator and operator of the technology in this fictionalized situation have a compassionate purpose? On one hand, Microsoft creator Bill Gates said, "Technology is unlocking the innate compassion we have for our fellow human beings" (Gates 2013). An interesting thought. On the other hand, the Dalai Lama said, "I think technology really increased human ability. But technology cannot produce compassion" (Almendrala 2014). The editors and authors of this book see in these remarks a dated dichotomy. It is not a simple competition of human versus machine. We believe that a compassionate healthcare system is one in which gifted humans and the best technologies collaborate to create exceptional, compassionate care.

As technology advances relentlessly, even rapaciously, healthcare is transforming radically. This book is therefore a call to action. We call upon healthcare professionals, leaders, educators, policy-makers, patients, and families to act: to shape a future in which healthcare is effective, accessible, efficient, and also fully anchored in compassion.

NOTE

1   I use the word *medical* in the broadest sense to indicate the field of practice of medicine and all the health professionals engaged in it. For the specific role of medical doctor I use the term *physician* to avoid confusion, as health professionals of many kinds have a doctoral degree (PhD or DPhil) and may use the title *Doctor*.

PART ONE

Coming to Terms with Compassion

I

Caring in a Digital Age: Exploring the Interface of Humans and Machines in the Provision of Compassionate Healthcare

David Wiljer, Gillian Strudwick, and Allison Crawford

INTRODUCTION

The term *compassion* derives from the Latin roots of "being with" (*cum* = with) and "suffering" (*passus, patior* = to suffer): being with one who is suffering. Understood this way, digital technologies may seem antithetical to compassion. As Hodges suggests in the introduction to this book, technologies can introduce new spaces between patients and carers, disrupting the human connection that constitutes compassionate care. And yet, if those who are suffering are inhabiting digital ecosystems, then understanding the meaning of compassion in the context of these evolving environments is critical for the quality of our health systems.

We are already inhabiting such ecosystems. The practice of healthcare has shifted from an experience that was primarily face to face and paper-based to a world dominated by digital tools, including electronic communications, decision-support tools, health information systems (e.g., electronic medical records and medication order entry), and remote patient encounters (through mobile apps, tele-consults, and virtual visits). Emerging technologies have further potential to transform how healthcare is delivered and who, or what, will deliver it. Technologies such as big data, AI, and machine learning may not even be visible to clinicians, though they could significantly affect the type of care patients receive and the outcomes achieved. Popular media has generated meaningful public debate on these topics, featuring provocative questions such as, "Will your clinicians be replaced by a robot?" (Sevunts 2017). What is the future of compassionate care in an environment dominated by technologies designed for patient safety, cost savings, and efficiency?

New technologies and digital care have profoundly affected the roles of patients, providers, and organizations, along with the design of care systems (Wiljer, Charow, et al. 2019). Although a great deal of research has examined the effects of new technologies and digital care, many questions remain (Keasberry, Scott, et al. 2018). Fundamental elements of care, such as equity of access, patient and provider satisfaction, usability, and resource utilization are rarely reported (Keasberry, Scott, et al. 2018). Compassion is often entirely absent from discussions of the impact of digital health on care delivery.

The digitalization of healthcare undoubtedly affects the means and ends of compassionate care. Digital tools may introduce new barriers, distractions, and distances that prevent healthcare providers from "being with" people in their care. At the same time, the promise of automation is, in part, to liberate clinicians to spend more time with their patients. The digital world can also create conduits to caring, enabling healthcare providers to be present with patients in new ways. These conduits may create new challenges and dilemmas, not only for frontline clinicians but also for organizations and healthcare delivery systems.

Some pioneering work has begun to delineate the concept of digital empathy (Powell and Roberts 2017; Terry and Cain 2016), while the impact of digital environments on compassion is still a new frontier for research. Many questions are just starting to surface. Fundamentally, how do we define digital compassion and understand compassion in a digital context? Do technologies simply mediate traditional experiences of compassion, or do they create new mechanisms for expressing compassion? How do we understand new forms and expressions of compassion and their effects on care? How do we shape our practices and policies to enable compassion? How do we prepare clinicians, patients, and their families to engage in such digitally enabled compassionate responses? Do digital technologies foster compassion by increasing access to care, or do they increase access at the expense of compassionate therapeutic relationships?

If we do not explore these issues and have open conversations, we run the risk that healthcare will be defined by technology and not by the humans who use it. Transformations can and should be collective and deliberate. They should be embedded in the design of new technologies and digital environments rather than being imposed by the necessity of finding efficiencies in an overburdened healthcare system.

This chapter examines how compassion can be expressed or impeded when care is delivered through digital means or in digital environments. We argue for an ecological approach to consider how technologies affect compassionate care. This approach directs our attention to the interrelationships among individuals, organizations, communities, and systems. The chapter has four main parts. The first part defines our terms and introduces the ecological approach. The second presents a framework for examining intersections between digital tools and compassionate responses. The third applies this approach to interactions between providers and patients, asking what is required of the compassionate "digital healthcare provider." The fourth applies the approach more broadly to organizations, communities, and systems, raising key issues such as trust, privacy, confidentiality, and cybersecurity. Scenarios are interspersed throughout the chapter to ground the conversation in situations that we all might experience.

Scenario 1: A Digitally Mediated Interaction

A therapist is seeing a client with intense suicidal ideation and worsening social isolation from family, friends, and the care team. During several sessions, the client reveals to the therapist that his suicidal ideation increases at night when he is alone. The therapist begins to worry about the client in the evenings and often has trouble falling asleep because of concern for the client's well-being. One evening, the therapist sends the client a text that reads, "Okay?" The client responds, and the therapist assumes he is safe. She is able to stop worrying and fall asleep. The therapist begins to text the client regularly in the evening and then begins to reflect upon whether this is an appropriate therapeutic interaction.

At its core, this scenario illustrates a simple and apparently compassionate intervention: the therapist feels connected to the suffering that the client experiences and responds through digital channels with a caring text message. Assuming consent has been given to communicate in this fashion, the interaction may seem rather benign. The therapist reaches out using a common technology and an everyday form of digital communication. Text messaging has been explored as a digital tool to enhance healthcare in several global contexts. For example, Lester, Ritvo, et al. (2010) published an important study in the *Lancet* demonstrating that people who received simple text messages had higher rates of adherence to antiretroviral treatment than those who did not. This approach to medication adherence has been replicated in other countries and contexts (Guo, Xu, et al. 2018). Thus, as a medium, text messages have shown potential to impact outcomes. The context and purpose in scenario 1, however, are substantially different. The therapist extends the therapeutic relationship from a physical setting to a digital one. Is this interaction appropriate? Is it safe for the client? Could it lead to distress and perhaps burnout for the therapist? The questions raised by this scenario are becoming fundamental to current practice in many settings. They illustrate dilemmas of digital professionalism that will help us to better understand the notion of digital compassion.

SECTION I: DIGITAL HEALTH
AND COMPASSIONATE CARE

Compassion is not simply a unidirectional flow from one provider/benefactor to one patient/recipient. It is interpersonal and multidirectional at the dyadic (patient-provider), team, and even institutional levels. Examining the dynamics of compassionate care, therefore, requires consideration of multiple sites and relationships. Similarly, *technology* itself is a heterogeneous category – one that continually evolves. Different types of technologies and digital tools have different effects on the therapeutic alliance and the delivery and outcomes of care. To understand these varied effects, it is essential to consider the context in which the technologies are used. The intersections of technology and compassion must be considered at multiple levels of the healthcare ecosystem, as illustrated in table 1.1. Each level draws attention to different dimensions of the ecosystem that can influence compassionate care.

Digital tools can affect compassionate care at the individual level by shaping actions, processes, attitudes, expectations, beliefs, and behaviours. The individual could be a healthcare professional, the patient or client, or a family member. Their understanding and

Table 1.1
Levels of the healthcare ecosystem

Individual digital provider	Dyad of patient and provider	Organization/ Institution	Community/ Society
Beliefs	Access to services	Leadership style	Values
Preferences	Communication	Patient, family and stakeholder involvement	Laws
Values	Therapeutic alliance		Social and health equity
Experiences	Health literacy	Policies	
Education	Digital literacy	Strategies	Perspectives on health and healing
Skills	Determinants of health	Budgets and resources	Perspectives on compassion and technology
Competencies			
Self-reflective capacity	Existing models of care	Implementation	
Personal ethics	Cultural beliefs and attitudes	Human resources and hiring practices	
Professional ethics		Education	
		Technology infrastructure and support	
		Data ownership	
		Privacy and storage	

experience of compassionate care can be substantially changed by the introduction of digital tools into the care environment. For example, health information and patient communities on the internet have given rise to the notion of the "e-patient" or expert patient. This concept changes the expectations that patients have of themselves and their providers. Rather than being passive participants, expert patients are active, engaged members of the team (HealthIt.gov 2015; Hoch and Ferguson 2005; Okun and Caligtan 2016). The evolution of the e-patient has brought expectations that care should be provided when and where it is needed, at any time of convenience and in ways that change the locus of control and power of decision-making (Okun and Caligtan 2016).

These shifting expectations significantly impact relationships. At the next level, the introduction of digital tools can transform the dynamic between the patient and provider. In the case of our first scenario, for example, the use of simple text messaging extends the spatial and temporal boundaries of the relationship. Digital tools may also affect how patients relate to their families and support systems or how health professionals relate to other members of an interprofessional team (Rashotte, Varpio, et al. 2016; Varpio, Day, et al. 2015). The changing digital system fundamentally changes the expectations of patients, requiring certain levels of health and digital literacy. At the same time, it changes models of care, available services, and the way the therapeutic relationship is expressed and experienced.

It is not sufficient to explore the notion of digital compassion at the individual level or even at the dyadic level. We must also consider the organization, community, and systems factors that shape the interface between digital environments and patients' experiences. These various factors will determine the ability of the ecosystem to support and foster digital compassion.

Little research has investigated how compassion is informed by healthcare environments (Christiansen, O'Brien, et al. 2015) or how organizational structures and processes can facilitate compassionate care (Crawford, Brown, et al. 2014). Compassion is often understood as a mental or behavioural state, prompting a focus on the individual characteristics and training of practitioners (Zamanzadeh, Valizadeh, et al. 2018). However, recent inquiry has begun to identify organizational and systemic facilitators and barriers to compassionate care. For example, organizational imperatives to standardize care, reduce costs, and improve efficiency may sometimes work at cross purposes to compassionate care. Moving away from blaming individual clinicians for lack of compassion toward recognizing these organizational or systemic pressures and constraints is essential for addressing barriers to compassionate care (Crawford, Brown, et al. 2014). Crawford (2011) has advanced the concept of the "organizational design" of compassionate care to encompass this underdeveloped domain. Similarly, Tierney, Seers, et al. (2017) find that individual desire and intention to provide compassionate care were insufficient. Compassionate care has to be realized within the "compassionate care flow" of an organization (Tierney, Seers, et al. 2017). It is within this complex ecosystem of relationships, from individual to system, that we can begin to understand and explore the emerging notion of digital compassion.

Technology is a broad term that in common discourse encompasses the application of new or innovative principles, knowledge processes, tools, and skills to solve problems (*Merriam-Webster* 2004; *Wikipedia* 2018). As Franklin (1999) argues, technology is about practice, the way we are organized to work and relate to one another, going beyond materials and extending into procedures, symbols, language, equations, and mindset. (See Paton and colleagues in chapter

3 of this book for further discussion of technologies as practice.) The notion of technology can also have a connotation of advancement and progress with the intention of improving the current state.

Healthcare providers increasingly work in digital and technology-laden clinical environments (Needleman 2013; Coiera 2015). Numerous technologies are currently available and will be present in healthcare settings in the future. These include a range of technologies at various stages of widespread adoption. *Electronic medical records (EMRs) and related digital tools* are patient-specific medical records accessible by healthcare providers (Chang and Gupta 2015) to support care quality and patient safety, including computerized order entry, barcode medication administration, electronic medication administration records, clinical decision-support systems, and risk flags. *Patient portals* are electronic platforms that allow patients (and sometimes family members) to access part or all of their EMR, to book appointments, or to communicate with a healthcare provider via messages (HealthIt.gov 2015). *Smart infusion pumps* are medical devices that regulate the rate of the intravenous delivering medications, hydration, or nutrition. These devices can be programmed with safety-specific information such as medication and flow rate. *Wearables* include technologies that can be worn and that track or log a certain function, such as sleep and activity. Care can also be delivered through *telehealth* to provide clinical care at a distance and through *mobile health* applications (Wozney 2017). Many other technologies exist within the healthcare context and/or with health applications such as robots, voice-activated assistants, social networking sites for people with similar conditions, and video games.

In the past few decades, the use of these technologies to enhance the delivery of care has been commonly described as eHealth. In 2005, a systematic review suggested that definitions of eHealth focused on how technology could be used to improve the processes of healthcare and address issues related to access, cost, quality, and portability of services (Oh, Rizo, et al. 2005). The notion of eHealth as a mechanism for collaboration, communication, and connection was an emergent, rather than a dominant, theme (Oh, Rizo, et al. 2005).

The definition of eHealth has continued to evolve. In 2014, Murray (2014) describes three types of eHealth interventions: (1) directly delivered interventions to patients or the public, which tend to focus on health promotion or enhancing self-management skills; (2) practice-level interventions, which focus on improving efficiency and meeting demand; and (3) tools for decision-makers to assess effectiveness and quality of care. In Murray's (2014, 326) conceptualization, eHealth is "not an operational extra: it is an essential part of cost-effective health service that offers high quality of care." Although these interventions may be effective, the primary drivers of use often include achieving operational efficiencies and meeting increased demand for service (Murray 2014).

The language of *digital health* is quickly replacing the language of eHealth and other related terms. Digital health is a term that has broader implications than a set of technologies used in the delivery of healthcare. Digital health has been defined as "the cultural transformation of how disruptive technologies that provide digital and objective data accessible to both caregivers and patients leads to an equal level doctor-patient relationship with shared decision-making and the democratization of care" (Meskó, Drobni, et al. 2017). This definition may overpromise the potential impact of digital health, but it illustrates that the idea of digital health extends far beyond the implementation of tools, processes, or data sets. It suggests a fundamental transformation of how care is delivered and received. Disruptive technologies may produce experiences that are difficult to recognize as healthcare, in the same way that communication has been transformed from the era of the telephone to the era of smart phone technologies and the ecosystems they engender. Furthermore, as Meskó, Dobni, et al. (2017) emphasize, digital health transforms the most basic healthcare relationship: the patient-provider relationship. Such transformation can be expected to affect fundamental processes, including decision-making and compassionate care.

The idea of compassion is often applied broadly, and at times can be used interchangeably with other emotions such as sympathy and empathy. What is the difference then between empathy and compassion for the purposes of this discussion? *Empathy* is often used as a broader term. According to Goetz and Simon-Thomas (2017, 6), "empathy can be pan-affective; people perceive, mirror and 'catch' all kinds of emotions, including amusement, pride, anger or sorrow." As Batson (quoted in Seppälä, Simon-Thomas, et al. 2017, 28) states, "empathetic concern ... is not a single, discrete emotion but includes a whole constellation of emotions. It includes feelings that people report as *sympathy, compassion, softheartedness, tenderness, sorrow, sadness, upset, distress, grief,* and more." Empathy, therefore, captures a range of emotional responses or feelings of being moved by the experiences of others. Within a digital healthcare ecosystem, the notion of empathy is helpful for exploring a broad range of emotional responses that can be experienced. Yet, the idea of empathy does not necessarily imply a corresponding action, intention, or agency.

Exploring the idea of digital compassion may in fact help us advance the conversation considerably by focusing on active and intentional responses to those feelings. "Compassion is a specific response to suffering ... [E]mpathy alone lacks a specific social urge, while compassion expressly involves feeling concerned and wanting to do something about it" (Goetz and Simon-Thomas 2017, 6). Goetz and Simon-Thomas (2017, 6) delineate multiple specific components of a compassionate response: (1) awareness of another's experience of suffering or need, (2) feeling "moved," (3) appraising one's own social role and abilities within the context of the suffering, (4) making judgments about the person who is suffering and their situational context, and (5) feeling driven to help.

These distinct components suggest specific mechanisms by which the emotional response of compassion may be translated into action. These mechanisms of action provide concrete links between the feelings one may experience and the actions one may take. Subsequent chapters in this book articulate clearly that every definition of compassion is only a partial definition with its own set of biases and limitations, and therefore continuous reflection is required (see chapter 6 by Paton and colleagues). This reminder is particularly important in the context of this discussion framed by one definition of compassion; because technologies are continually evolving, constant and critical reflection on the relationship between emerging technologies and the delivery of compassionate care will be necessary. Recognizing the limitations and emergent nature of this lens on compassion, we will consider in the remainder of the chapter how this proposed mechanism may be translated or transformed within the context of digital healthcare.

SECTION 2. INTERSECTION OF
DIGITAL TOOLS AND COMPASSIONATE CARE

We shall consider how digital technologies might mediate each component of compassionate care described above. Digital tools may shape the experience of compassion in healthcare in various ways by: (1) raising awareness of suffering; (2) mediating emotional responses to suffering; (3) creating new means of responding; (4) providing a platform for education, coaching, and training around compassionate care in the digital ecosystem; (5) enabling compassionate

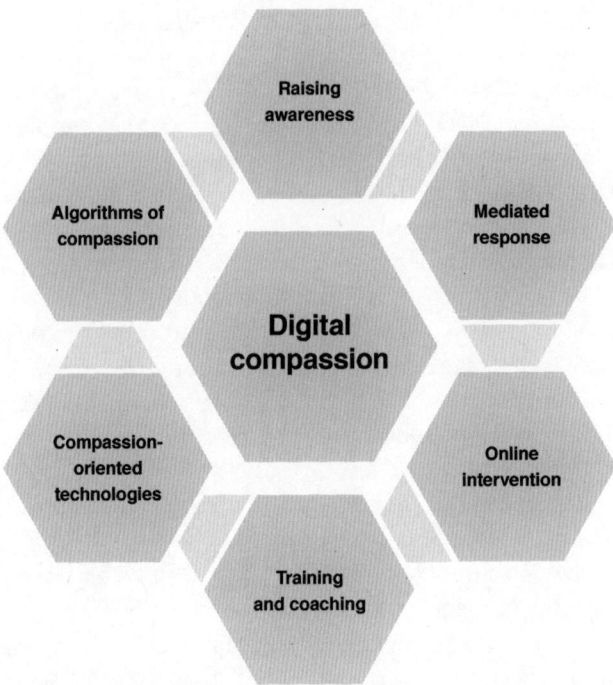

Figure 1.1 Digital intersections with compassionate care

actions; and (6) simulating or automating compassionate responses (Kemp, Zhang, et al. 2020) (see figure 1.1).

It is important to note these are fluid categories that are interrelated and not mutually exclusive. The intention of this section is not to create rigid categories of technology but rather to establish a common language that can, to a certain extent, be mapped to our working definition of compassion. The elements of this definition are themselves fluid; they represent distinct but not linear or sequential components of compassionate responses. The examples given below are, therefore, illustrative and could be applied to several elements and points of intersection.

The first component of compassion is building awareness of another's experience of suffering or need. The ability of digital media to create awareness of suffering is perhaps best illustrated by the well-known photograph of a young Syrian boy, Alan Kurdi, who was found lying dead on a beach in 2015 (Kingsley and Timur 2015). The image went viral and led to a global shift in the awareness of the Syrian refugee crises, which in turn led to a global empathetic outpouring. More importantly, it led to compassionate and real change in individual behaviours, organizational structures, and government policy. However, this mechanism of digital media to create awareness about human suffering is not without its challenges and limitations. Many have raised questions about the potential to bombard and ultimately anaesthetize us to suffering, or to make us passive consumers or voyeurs of the suffering of others.

Digital tools have also been used to build awareness within healthcare systems. Social media has been used, for example, to raise public awareness around mental health issues. Popular campaigns such as Bell Let's Talk Day have used the power of digital technologies to raise awareness around issues of mental health across an entire country and to generate conversations around important social and health topics. The purpose of Bell Let's Talk is to encourage conversations to raise awareness and money to help eliminate stigma related to mental illness. The campaign has reported fostering over 867 million interactions since 2011 (Bell Let's Talk 2019), resulting in significant new funding for the mental health community. Within the healthcare field, there are many successful examples of digital tools used to raise awareness of the suffering of others. While the potential to disseminate misinformation or to engage in socially unproductive behaviour is always present, digital tools can contribute to the first step of compassion in creating "awareness of another's experience of suffering or need" (Seppälä, Simon-Thomas, et al. 2017).

The examples above illustrate how digital tools can bring suffering to the attention of wider audiences; they make suffering visible, allowing us to witness the experiences of others. In the process, they can also shape the nature of our emotional responses and judgments. For example, the photographs of Alan Kurdi sharply invoked for many of us our own experiences. The toddler was pictured alone, fully dressed, face down in the sand at the water's edge. We could relate personally to the tragic scene in ways that moved us to respond.

At the same time, we can become hypersaturated by images of suffering that we feel powerless to prevent. Images may be designed not to invoke compassion toward others but rather to invoke resentment, fear, or blame. Digital media, therefore, may raise awareness while inhibiting our capacity to feel or to act upon compassionate responses. In the context of the digital health ecosystem, it may often be helpful to differentiate the more passive use of technology in raising awareness of suffering from the intentional design and use of digital tools to deliberately create a positive, action-oriented response to that awareness.

In healthcare, the notion of mediated responses is perhaps best illustrated by the movement of digital storytelling. At its core, digital storytelling involves telling patient stories in digital formats in order to create connections and conversations (Sanchez-Laws 2010). Hardy and Sumner (2018), in their book *Cultivating Compassion: How Digital Storytelling is Transforming Healthcare*, chronicle fifteen years of experience in developing the Patient Voices Programme (www. patientvoices.org.uk) to drive change in healthcare. Patient Voices has developed a consistent and comprehensive approach to integrating digital stories to build critical consciousness and social awareness (Hardy and Sumner 2018). Through a process that involves both a workshop and the creation of the stories, the program has created initiatives to support change in numerous areas, including mental health, dementia, COPD, and arthritis. It has also created initiatives to influence organizational cultures and to highlight important systems issues across the National Health Service in the United Kingdom. By focusing on the human elements of healthcare, digital storytelling can be integrated into the process of educating and motivating individuals, organizations, and systems to recognize suffering and formulate a judgment that a response is required.

Technology and digital tools present an enormous opportunity to support compassionate approaches to care through education, training, and coaching. Online training has the potential to build capacity and expertise among clinicians to deliver compassionate care using digital technologies. For example, online courses and modules can be used to ensure that trainees and health professionals can effectively deliver compassionate care through telemedicine. Online tools can also be used to share and disseminate best practices. For instance, communities of practice could be established to ensure that clinicians have a forum to share knowledge and build a collective expertise around the effective use of digital tools to deliver compassionate care to patients and their families. In addition to mediating compassionate responses, digital storytelling is also a powerful educational practice. Howkins and Hardy used digital storytelling to develop an interprofessional education program on palliative care (Hardy and Sumner 2018). As we provide care in an environment driven by technologies and digital tools, we must prepare professionals to use these tools to deliver care that is not just effective and efficient but also compassionate. Curricula around digital professionalism are emerging in many training programs. These curricula should include competencies specific to digital compassion (Ellaway, Coral, et al. 2015).

The ability for healthcare providers to use digital tools and technologies to deliver care in a compassionate way will vary based on the technology and its function or purpose. Health professionals and providers will need to determine how a particular technology or digital tool can be integrated in their workflow, and whether the technology can be used during the clinical encounter in a meaningful way. Ensuring that healthcare providers are equipped with the appropriate knowledge and skills to adopt these technologies meaningfully is essential to the delivery of compassionate care now and in the future.

Healthcare providers will also need to assess their patients' attitudes toward specific technologies and tailor their use accordingly (Booth 2016; Griffin, Skinner, et al. 2016; Lane 2018). Not all patients will perceive a technology or digital tool in the same way. For example, a recent study found that patients have different perceptions of barcode scanning technology used to improve the safety of medication administration. Whereas some patient participants said that this technology made them feel the healthcare provider cared about them, others reported the process of scanning their hospital wristband made them feel objectified, like an item in the grocery store (Strudwick, Clark, et al. 2017). In this case, the use of technology enhanced the perception of patient-centred care for some, while it detracted from the therapeutic relationship for others. Thus there is an emerging need to integrate principles of compassionate care into the design and implementation of these tools. Digital approaches can also be used to provide care in a timely fashion in regions or populations that might not have access to other methods of providing services. In these cases, using digital tools may become a mechanism for mediating a compassionate response in a timely fashion, if these tools are designed and implemented with the principles of providing compassionate care in mind.

As decision-support and AI technologies become more mature, digital tools will draw heavily on automation and algorithmic responses in the delivery of care. Decision-support tools – such as alerts, order sets, templated care plans and forms, clinical pathways and chatbots – are used increasingly to standardize best practices in care and offer guidance to healthcare providers. Often embedded within electronic medical records (EMRs) and order entry systems, these tools alert healthcare providers of potentially pertinent information required for decision-making and care, such as a patient allergy to a medication that is ordered. One of the challenges of these algorithms is their rigidity and thus their lack of person-specific recommendations. Healthcare providers may become frustrated with these systems if suggestions are not specific enough to the needs of their patients. Additionally, the frequency of alerts in modern-day systems often cause alert fatigue and may add to technology-induced burnout.

As digital ecosystems further integrate AI, algorithms, and automation into care delivery, there will be an opportunity to assimilate Artificial Emotional Intelligence (AEI) into the delivery of healthcare. Garg, Singhal, et al. (n.d., n.p.) report how they have integrated AI and AEI to "study and develop systems that recognize, interpret, process and simulate human emotions." AEI uses algorithms and affective computing to identify relevant emotions; recognize, express, and model emotions; and develop responses. Other AI experts are exploring the potential for multi-modal inputs to make AI emotionally intelligent. These include, for example, facial measurements and tone of voice (Krakovsky 2018).

AEI may have the capacity to respond to situations using simulated empathetic responses, but little is known about how these responses will be perceived and how they will impact the experience of care. Daugherty and Wilson (2018, 117), in their book *Human + Machine: Reimagining Work in the Age of* AI, describe a potential new role for human work: the empathy trainer, "an individual who will teach AI systems to display compassion." They have identified the emergent need for individuals who will train AI to have more empathetic responses in a variety of situations. Companies such as Koko, a spinoff of MIT Media Lab, are developing systems that help service-oriented chatbots to have deeper sympathetic and emotional responses (Daugherty and Wilson 2018). The possibility is quite real that these new roles will emerge soon.

As these technologies develop, they may transform our notion of compassion. At a minimum, there is a need for conversation and reflection on whether AEI has a place in the future of healthcare and the future of compassionate care. However, healthcare providers need to apply critical thinking to these new technologies and processes to avoid passively accepting suggestions generated through technologies that could cause harm to patients.

SECTION 3. DIGITAL HEALTHCARE
PROVIDERS AND COMPASSIONATE CARE

Many healthcare professionals have not been trained to provide care, and specifically compassionate care, in a digital environment. In this section, we consider how healthcare professionals can become competent, compassionate, and confident in using digital tools. We use the term *digital healthcare provider* to describe any health professional who is trained to deliver patient-centred care using the available digital tools and technologies, inclusive of understanding the security and privacy of digital information, the positioning and use of technology in the clinical encounter, and other relevant topics. The digital healthcare provider will also be able to apply these principles to new and emerging digital tools and technologies and to adapt their use of these tools according to patient need, comfort, and preference.

We begin with an example that illustrates how technologies can compromise compassionate care. We then use this example to explore some intricacies of establishing and maintaining a therapeutic relationship in digital healthcare environments.

Scenario 2: Technology and the Clinical Encounter
An elderly couple, Mary and Gordon, have lived in their home for over thirty years in a small rural community. The couple regularly visit a nurse practitioner in their community primary care centre. Recently, they have visited more frequently due to increasingly complex health-related needs. The primary care centre has been present in the community for nearly fifty years and has recently implemented an EMR system for patient information to be documented and stored digitally. A desktop computer has been installed in each examination room for the nurse practitioner to access the EMR, even though the rooms were not built to accommodate such hardware.

Thus, when Mary and Gordon arrive for their medical appointment they both notice that the presence of the computer in addition to the people make the examination room feel crowded. During their visit, the nurse practitioner constantly turns away from them to type notes into the record and to look up information. Consequently, a significant portion of the interaction is completed with the nurse practitioner's back turned toward the couple. Although the couple is unable to see the information displayed on the computer screen, they can tell the nurse practitioner is frustrated when they hear, "It won't let me go to the next page." At the end of the interaction, the couple express to one another that the computer was the focus of attention. They worry that they were not heard and wonder whether the plan of care determined with the nurse practitioner will sufficiently meet their complex health needs.

In the above scenario, a primary care clinic has implemented a technology (an EMR and related hardware) in an effort to improve patient care. However, several challenges arise in the use of this technology that negatively influence the clinical interaction between the elderly couple and the nurse practitioner. First, the room is not large enough to comfortably accommodate the technology along with the patients and provider. It is therefore unsurprising that the couple feel discomfort when they first encounter the new technology. Second, the position of the computer in the room creates a challenging environment to effectively communicate. The nurse practitioner has to turn away from the couple, so that they are unable to see what he is doing, leading them to question whether they were heard. Finally, the nurse practitioner has difficulties using the technology and is therefore distracted from the clinical encounter. These difficulties could be due to various factors related to training, usability of the system, or software malfunctions. Regardless of the reason, the technology detracts from the delivery of compassionate person-centred care.

This scenario need not play out in the practice environments of today or in the future. Effective digital healthcare providers can ensure that technology is used in meaningful and beneficial ways to deliver person-centred healthcare. They can also work with healthcare organizations to select and implement technologies that can be used effectively and compassionately with and for patients.

The therapeutic relationship between a healthcare provider and a patient is the cornerstone of compassionate care (Cole and McLean 2003). It is a purposeful relationship directed toward the goal of advancing the best interest of and outcome for the client (Stickley and Freshwater 2008). Given that technology may be used as a communication conduit, or is used to support data collection and decision-making, the following questions may be asked: What happens to this therapeutic relationship when digital tools and technologies are used in the delivery of care? Can a therapeutic relationship be established using technology? There is likely no uniform answer to these questions, since personal factors (e.g., comfort with technology), type of technology, and the way in which technology is used all play a significant role in how technology is perceived and how it affects the therapeutic relationship (Strudwick 2015). We consider these factors below.

Healthcare providers and patients alike are not equally adept and comfortable using the various technologies available within healthcare settings (Holden 2012). Exposure to technology outside of the healthcare context may influence both groups' attitudes toward the use of technology for healthcare-related purposes (Strudwick, Clark, et al. 2018). If and when possible, healthcare providers need to assess the comfort level of their patients and tailor their use of the technology accordingly. For example, if a patient is comfortable with viewing their EMR, the healthcare provider may want to explain what they are looking for in the record, and what they are writing, while showing the screen to the patient. For other patients who are less comfortable, the documentation could be left until the face-to-face encounter has been completed, if possible. Similarly, patients' attitudes and access should also be assessed before making any decisions to use technology exclusively for a particular reason. For example, if educational materials are made available via a website, they may also need to be made available in another form (e.g., paper) so that people without access to the internet are not inadvertently excluded.

Several articles have been written about the use of EMRs in the clinical encounter (Duffy, Fochtmann, et al. 2016; Lanier, Dao, et al. 2017; Mickan, Atherton, et al. 2014; Street, Liu, et al. 2017). In a recent study, physicians were observed interacting with patients while also using an EMR system (Street, Liu, et al. 2017). Findings of this study showed that patients became less participative when their physicians were typing more frequently during the interaction. Similarly, when physicians looked at the computer more often, there was more silence during the clinical interaction. These findings suggest that healthcare providers should be mindful of how much typing they are doing and where they are looking during the clinical encounter. Healthcare providers need to demonstrate that they are engaged in the conversation with the patient, using the EMR as a tool to support care.

Increasing attention is being paid to understanding and promoting effective practices for using digital tools at the point of care. Fleischmann, Duhm, et al. (2015) conducted a study to determine if the introduction of tablets during ward rounds would decrease the amount of time physicians spent completing the medical record, in comparison to a computer-based record system. Findings of this study suggested that the tablet, rather than the computer, better supported physician workflow, allowing physicians to spend more time at the bedside with patients and less time completing the medical record. Although tablets may be a viable option for some healthcare providers, further investigation is needed to analyze whether they can be feasibly incorporated into various workflows. As healthcare providers generally value spending time with their patients, identifying ways that technology can be leveraged to provide additional time, rather than competing for time, would be of value.

Through these types of studies, best practices are starting to emerge, including: (1) point to the screen and show patients what is typed; (2) actively look at the patient and not the technology; (3) begin the interaction by talking to the patient and then bring in the technology; and (4) tell patients why technology is used. Healthcare provider use of technology within their practice has brought about many improvements to care; however, careful attention must be paid to how they use the technology during clinical encounters with patients to ensure that therapeutic communication is maintained.

Substantial efforts have been made to incorporate education on the use of digital technologies into medicine, nursing, and pharmacy programs in Canada, and to ensure that knowledgeable faculty are available to teach this subject (Canada Health Infoway 2018a; Canada Health Infoway 2018b; Crawford, Sunderji, et al. 2017; Sunderji, Crawford, and Jovanovic 2015). However, since education about the use of digital technologies is relatively new in healthcare provider entry-to-practice programs, several challenges have arisen. One challenge is that most healthcare providers currently practicing have not received this education and thus may not hold the appropriate digital technology competencies to allow them to practice in compassionate and patient-centred ways. Faculty members often lack the digital health competencies needed to teach this content to students. Finally, once practicing, healthcare providers have limited opportunities to obtain formal education or training with regard to using digital technologies in compassionate and person-centred ways. Thus, there is an opportunity to further develop education and training programs to support healthcare provider students, educators, and those currently practicing. Digital tools and the digital ecosystem also offer unique opportunities to provide training to help digital healthcare providers develop their skills as new technologies emerge.

In scenario 2 described previously, the presence of technology led the nurse practitioner to be less present during the interaction, which resulted in the patients questioning whether they had been truly heard, and whether their care needs had been appropriately met. This scenario may have had the opposite effect had the nurse practitioner been more aware of how to meaningfully use technology with this couple, through acting as a digital healthcare provider. For example, the digital provider could advocate for hardware that was more appropriately sized for the physical space. They could acknowledge the presence of the technology, describe the options for using it, and ask the couple their preferences. The computer screen could have been positioned such that everyone in the examination room could view the content, and the digital healthcare provider could have explained what information they were adding to the record. The provider could have received an appropriate level of training and practice with the technology before using it with patients, avoiding potentially challenging moments during patient interactions.

If the nurse practitioner acted effectively as a digital healthcare provider, the couple may have left the appointment feeling they were listened to, their needs were addressed, and their health was deemed important enough to warrant the use of sophisticated technologies. This scenario also points to challenges that go beyond ensuring we have digital health professionals. Organizations and systems must also be re-examined and reimagined to enable digital health professionals to thrive.

SECTION 4. DIGITAL HEALTH SYSTEMS AND COMPASSIONATE CARE

Interpersonal relationships between providers, patients, and their families remain foundational to compassionate care, but in order to flourish, digital compassion needs advancement at an organizational and health systems level. Compassion requires a collaborative effort and is shaped by social and cultural influences, including programmatic, institutional, and systems factors. Similarly, technology is situated within networks of patients and providers that extend outside organizations and institutions. This section focuses on practical strategies that organizations can use to assess their current approach to digital compassion and to support compassionate care across all programs and environments that employ technology and digital tools.

Organization-level barriers to providing compassionate care include lack of values or missions centred on compassionate care; policies that promote an individualistic approach, such as individual practitioner accountability and training; lack of a systematic, thoughtful approach to compassionate design; an organizational culture of threat or blame; healthcare business models that focus inappropriately on "turnaround" and efficiency of patient discharge; time and resource constraints; heavy workloads; and inadequate staffing levels (Christiansen, O'Brien, et al. 2015; Tierney, Seers, et al. 2017; Valizadeh, Zamanzadeh, et al. 2018).

Organizations can also create environments and implement strategies that enable compassionate care to thrive. Tierney, Seers, et al. (2017) found that organizations with good "compassionate care flow" were explicit in their intention to improve patient health and the role of providers through compassion. Compassionate organizations articulate values and vision around compassion, and adopt practices to support these values throughout the organization (Ramage, Curtis, et al. 2017). Compassionate organizations also have compassionate leaders who provide positive role modelling, facilitate a collective team identity, and foster a community where all feel valued and supported (Christiansen, O'Brien, et al. 2015). (For further discussion of compassionate leadership, see chapter 6 of this book.)

Optimally, processes to assess and enhance compassion within a healthcare organization will be based on available evidence and implementation science. This work is in the early stages of development and maturity. Ramage, Curtis, et al. (2017) have developed a tool kit that addresses compassionate care at individual and organizational levels, including compassion indicators to assess leadership and organizational culture. Such promising efforts need to be validated in other settings. There is much to be learned from other systems- and practice-change initiatives, such as recent efforts to cultivate trauma-informed organizations. The Trauma Informed Organizational Checklist developed by Arthur, Seymour, et al. (2013), for example, has widely disseminated implementation strategies for overall policy and program mandate, leadership, hiring practices, training for staff, support and supervision of staff, screening and assessment, policies and procedures, and monitoring and evaluation. The Substance Abuse and Mental Health Services Administration in the United States also has a guide with implementation strategies to create trauma-informed organizations (MSI 2013).

Within the field of digital health, including eHealth and telehealth research, implementation and systems planning are even less developed (Wozney 2017; Serhal, Arena, et al. 2018; Serhal, Crawford, et al. 2017). Several authors have attempted to delineate implementation approaches. Serhal, Arena, et al. (2018), for example, use the Consolidated Framework for Implementation Research (Damschroder, Aron, et al. 2009), which includes factors related to the "inner setting," or organizational setting, such as culture and values, relative priority, organizational incentives, and feedback and learning climate. Attention to these factors can help assess an organization's readiness to adopt technologies. The same strategies could be used regarding factors related to readiness to adopt digital compassion as a value and priority. To our knowledge, compassionate care at an organizational level has not received adequate attention within digital movements and the deployment of many technologies.

Recent reports by the Mental Health Commission of Canada (2017) identified the need for greater implementation of science approach to advance digital health innovation (see also Wozney 2017). There is awareness of the importance of focusing on context, community, and cultural needs so that "appropriate technology can be defined as the easiest technological solution that achieves the desired purpose within the social, cultural, environmental and economic conditions of the setting in which it is to be applied" (Wozney 2017, 12). Cultural and community awareness requires solutions that "respect local traditions, expectations of the healthcare system, beliefs about health and disease, health literacy and usage patterns of existing healthcare services" (Wozney 2017, 12). Co-design with patients and families is one approach that can improve the relevance of digital interventions. While these approaches advance consideration of technology at an organizational level, none of them mentions compassionate care.

There are few guidelines and standards to ensure digital environments are designed to foster compassionate care. A vast array of standards pertaining to technical aspects, privacy, and implementation have been applied to digital technologies. For example, a seven-stage EMR adoption model has been developed by the Healthcare Information and Management Systems Society (HIMSS Analytics 2017). The stages of adoption focus on the implementation of tools that will promote digitally enabled care. However, these models do not assess the standard of care that is provided in those environments. Future work should explore the creation of *digital compassion standards* that clearly outline the types of experiences that digital environments will deliver. We also need policies and procedures that promote digital compassion. Such policies would improve the implementation of technology and perhaps help prevent staff burnout, which has recently been associated with the introduction of technologies such as electronic health records. (See the discussion by Maunder, Chaukos, and Lawson in chapter 4 of this book.) The question remains: What would digital compassion look like within a healthcare organization?

Scenario 4: Organizational Digital Compassion

Dr Metelsky is program director of a new hospital initiative in e-mental healthcare. The hospital's goal is to increase access to mental health services by seeing more clients and serving more of the smaller towns that surround their urban hospital. The CEO is excited about the project because it will enhance the hospital's reputation for innovation and expand the population served. An extensive strategic planning process results in a rewriting of the hospital mission and vision statements to highlight this new emphasis on innovation and access to healthcare. Resources are invested in setting up telehealth studios and in equipment. Twelve months later, the initiative is deemed a great success. Referrals to the hospital have increased by 200 per cent. The hospital hosts an innovation conference to highlight program successes. They are shocked when patients, families, and several community agencies show up to protest the telehealth program, citing concerns about lack of follow-up and about consultants who seem "impersonal" and know nothing about their community. Several physicians from surrounding communities are also angry because they feel displaced.

This example highlights the pitfalls of a focus on technology as a means to increase access without due attention to how the introduction of new tools and processes will impact the quality of care – including the patient, family, and community experience of care as compassionate. There is a mismatch in scenario 3 between the goals of the hospital and the needs and experiences of the community it serves. Technology can significantly disrupt the delivery and flow of care as well as relationships of care within a system. Technology cannot replace knowledge of culture and community. Unless a healthcare organization focuses on compassion as a core value, compassion will not be central to its offered services, including any delivered via technology. In this case, some of this discrepancy in aims and results could have been avoided through early and ongoing engagement with the community, perhaps extending to co-design, along with a focus on compassion as a core value alongside other outcomes, including increased access.

A compassionate organization demonstrates a commitment to compassionate practices and organizational reassessments, continually adjusting to patients' needs. Compassionate organizations incorporate technology into care in compassionate ways, and support compassion within healthcare encounters that occur within a digital environment. In chapter 7 of this book, Martimianakis and colleagues explore the principles that guide compassionate organizations. The following considerations complement their discussion, suggesting strategies that apply specifically to digital compassion:[1]

1   Commit to being a compassionate organization in all healthcare environments, including tele- and digital platforms. Strive for innovation with attention to quality, including compassion and safety.
2   Create an infrastructure to initiate, support, and guide compassion as a core part of the strategic development of eHealth.
3   Involve patients, families, and other external stakeholders who will engage with healthcare services via proposed technologies. In particular, consider marginalized populations within the institution and communities served.
4   Assess how the organization's current policies, procedures, operations, and digital tools or technologies either support or hinder compassionate care.
5   Develop a plan to implement and support compassion within eHealth programs, services, and platforms within the organization.
6   Implement quality improvement measures as needs and problem areas related to digital compassion are identified.
7   Reassess the implementation of the organizational plan and its ability to meet the needs of patients, families, and communities and to provide consistent digital compassionate care.
8   Institute practices that support sustainability of digital compassion, such as ongoing training; clinical supervision; patient, family, and community participation and feedback; and resource allocation.

As we develop organizations and systems that are responsible contributors to the digital ecosystem, the notions of trust and a trusted environment are key to creating a robust digital health ecosystem (Bertino, Khan, et al. 2006). Trust is the foundation for compassion and equally for digital compassion. Three elements are essential for establishing the trust required for digital compassion. The first is privacy. Privacy is a complex concept with many meanings and connotations, but in its simplest form, it is the ability of the individual to control the use of information that relates to them (Shen, Bernier, et al. 2019). This notion of privacy needs to be protected as part of digital compassion.

Second, confidentiality refers to the responsibility of healthcare professionals to safeguard personal health information within the circle of care. In the digital ecosystem, the parameters of the circle of care can become quite blurred. In a recent case in the United Kingdom, a hospital shared over a million identifiable records with an industry partner. Their intention was to improve the quality of patient care; however, patients did not consent directly to the terms of the data sharing (Powles and Hodson 2017). This action therefore reduced public trust. Ensuring good data governance is essential to establishing digital compassion.

Finally, healthcare providers and organizations are obligated to secure personal health information to ensure that unauthorized access or data breaches do not occur. With the recent rise of cybercrime, cybersecurity has become a priority safety issue for healthcare organizations. Organizations must protect themselves and their patients against cybercrimes and ensure that healthcare professionals have the knowledge, skills, and attitudes to promote cybersecurity (Kruse, Frederick, et al. 2017). Cybersecurity will emerge as an important element of digital compassion. As we have already seen, other ethical issues are also emerging. Individuals, organizations, and systems must attend to these issues to build the trust that will be required to promote digital compassion and compassionate care in the digital ecosystem.

CONCLUSION

Digital tools will significantly impact the nature of compassionate care. They may disrupt traditional relationships through the veil of technology or they may act as conduits of caring, supporting traditional relationships and creating new opportunities for meaningful compassionate care. These effects will likely vary with each particular type of technology, with their context of use, and with the perceptions of their users. They may be unpredictable, and they will certainly be dispersed across the digital health ecosystem. We will, therefore, need to be vigilant in attending to these effects to ensure that technologies serve, rather than threaten, the aim of compassionate care. In this chapter, we have taken some first steps toward articulating a framework for examining the different ways that technologies might mediate compassionate responses and translate those responses into action. We have also begun to envision how digital healthcare providers and digital healthcare organizations can adopt compassion as a central governing principle within digital healthcare environments.

In order to ensure that technologies add value to patient care, a concerted effort will be needed from healthcare providers and healthcare organizations alike, along with educators, designers, and researchers. It will be important to ensure that both patients and healthcare providers are involved in identifying the need for new technologies, as well as selecting, planning, implementing, using, and evaluating new technologies. At the same time, organizations and systems must adopt compassionate care as a central guiding principle in their development of digital health ecosystems.

NOTE

1   These strategies are adapted from the framework created for implementation of trauma-informed care.

2

Patient Engagement and Compassionate Care

Paula Rowland and Jennifer Johannesen

This book invites imagination. It asks us not merely to speculate about the future but to actively shape how the future of healthcare will unfold. We take up this challenge by turning to a declaration that now echoes through various health policy circles: The perspectives of healthcare providers, policy-makers, and administrators are impor-tant but insufficient for imagining the future of healthcare. Patients, family members, and caregivers have a vital role to play in shaping that imaginary.

This declaration leads us to a growing world of patient engage-ment.[1] Some might call it an industry. We refer here to a particular kind of patient engagement: programs usually initiated by healthcare organizations that invite current or past patients to share their experi-ences and insights with the stated aim of improving organizational practices, programs, or policies. The involvement of patients in this way shifts their role from that of subject (in a research context) to that of collaborator or partner. For example, patients might serve on long-standing committees, participate in single-day quality improve-ment events, speak at conferences, or provide information through interviews, focus groups, or other consultative exercises. Patients and healthcare professionals alike assume that these kinds of activities are valuable opportunities for patients to influence and improve healthcare practice.

As authors of this chapter, we both have direct experience with this world of patient engagement programs and practices, albeit from different standpoints, as we will describe. We have been invited to consider relationships between patient engagement practices and the aspiration of compassionate patient care, all within an increasingly technological landscape. In doing so, we found ourselves mapping what we already know about patient engagement practices, considering how these practices might connect to (and complicate) the concept of compassionate care, and wondering how these intersections might develop as technologies emerge. These questions required us to wrestle with big ideas – compassion, suffering, humanity – and how they are translated and transformed as they intersect with the practical realities of running patient engagement programs within healthcare organizations.

As co-authors, we have worked together often enough to identify and appreciate our points of agreement and divergence. We do not attempt to smooth over those divergences here. Indeed, we value these as opportunities to further deliberate on and to better understand each other's points of view. In doing so, we hope to enrich existing debate and perhaps uncover issues that were previously hidden or unexpressed. Ultimately, this process of deliberation allows us to better articulate what we agree on, what we can wonder about, and what our divergences imply, all of which are instrumental to tackling the challenging topic before us. We therefore begin, in the next section, by introducing ourselves and our respective relationships to the topics at hand. We then unpack several meanings of compassion, mapping them onto three distinct approaches to patient engagement.

LOCATING OURSELVES IN THIS CONVERSATION

Paula Rowland:
Researcher, Clinician, Earnest Advocate for "Better"

I started my career in healthcare as an occupational therapist. Working primarily with children and adults who had sustained some form of neurotrauma, I helped individuals and families rediscover their lives while experiencing minds and bodies drastically changed. Many people think occupational therapists help people return to work. And, of course, many occupational therapists do work in vocational rehabilitation settings. But occupational therapists conceive of occupation more broadly, to include all the ways we humans meaningfully occupy our time. This might include paid work, but it also includes the leisure pursuits that give us joy and the unpaid roles that are important in our lives, for example, as parents, siblings, friends, or students. As an occupational therapist, I helped a young mother who had a stroke learn how to change a squirmy toddler's diaper while using just one hand (not an easy feat!). I helped a teenage boy cast a fishing rod for the first time, months after a major car accident in Canada's North. I also helped countless people with invasive brain tumours find comfort in their last days of life.

In these moments of intimacy – moments of grief, resilience, anger, joy – I always felt privileged to be part of patients' and families' lives during some of their most vulnerable moments. This, I felt, was participating in something important. While I came to think much more critically about my own practice as a therapist, I could never imagine working anywhere other than healthcare.

I think because I've always been so enamoured with what healthcare could be that I felt almost personally hurt when I saw it fall short of my tenderly held ideals: When I saw my colleagues (or found myself!) being brash, rude, or unkind. When I saw patients and families get lost in overly hostile environments (why are hospitals so notoriously difficult to navigate?). Or when I felt stuck in absurd policies that seemed to serve the sole purpose of frustrating my abilities to provide compassionate care. A desire for things to be better animated my work as a young clinician and later as a healthcare leader. When I found myself as a family member accompanying loved ones in intensive care units, emergency departments, and palliative care rooms, well, I felt even sadder about all the ways I was confronted with the various fault lines in my field.

I still hold this desire for better. I believe that our healthcare people, practices, and places should not add to the burden of illness, and that continual improvement is a moral imperative. But I now approach these aims as a researcher. I use social science theories and approaches to help me unpack the various tensions, dilemmas, and complexities that will always occupy our attempts to improve. This includes asking questions about professional and institutional power, about voice and voicelessness, and about how these social and political dynamics work their way into determining who gets to do what and how authority and responsibility are distributed. I dig for unintended consequences of organizational initiatives, and I look for the unruly manifestations of neatly scribed policies and plans.

This is the researcher stance that I bring to my explorations of patient engagement programs. I approach these programs with great appreciation for the generosity, commitment, and effort that people bring to this work. And yet, I think my utmost opportunity for contribution is in approaching the task of research with some distance from the programs themselves. Distance enables me to converse with these programs while resisting the predefined, immutable position of either advocate or critic. By side-stepping the imposed binary between problem-solving and criticism, I hope to engage in a third space described eloquently by Alan Cribb (2018, 110): "On the one hand there is the ethical imperative to address the inadequacies of health policies and services, including the substantial harms that are caused by healthcare deficiencies. On the other hand, there is the less pressing but still practically relevant skeptical task of asking how well equipped we are to 'improve' things – how far we know what we are talking about and doing when we seek to be useful in this way. The debate between these two forms of moral seriousness is alive and well."

As a researcher, I'm an interlocutor between these two poles of moral seriousness. I maintain some distance from specific improvement programs because I want to give my best possible (always imperfect, always humble) contribution to the larger shared aspiration: continual striving toward better healthcare. This means balancing specific practical questions with more fundamental ones. How can specific patient engagement efforts help make healthcare more compassionate? But what is patient engagement? What are its limits and social functions? How might they serve or compromise care?

Jennifer Johannesen: Caregiver, "Engaged Patient," Bioethicist

I came to the topic of patient engagement quite by accident, although in hindsight it was perhaps inevitable. My own patient experience is that of caregiver. My son, Owen, was born with multiple severe disabilities, requiring full support for all aspects of daily living until he died at the age of twelve. I wrote about our experiences with healthcare, pediatric rehab, and special education in my book *No Ordinary Boy* (2011). It was through that process of writing and reflecting on our experiences that I came to see a common thread: many encounters with healthcare organizations that I had experienced as a parent seemed, in hindsight, both absurd and tragic. When I think about those encounters, the word *compassionate* does not come to mind. Instead, I recall endless bureaucracy, the need to be on my best behaviour, predetermined options represented as autonomous decisions. I remember an overwhelming sense of being *managed*. I was rewarded for calm rationality and praised for good behaviour. My class and cultural privilege awarded me respect that I worked hard to keep. I remember how stressful and tiring it was, trying to ensure we were always seen to be *deserving* of good care. Although my son received excellent medical care and I was typically treated respectfully, I continue to be amazed at how effectively – and invisibly – the structures and practices of healthcare organizations managed my experiences and behaviours in a way that optimized organizational efficiency, all the while making me feel like I was in control. This is one of the lenses through which I think about patient engagement.

Some time after Owen died and I had published my book, I wanted to immerse myself in theory and literature that both moved my attention beyond my personal story and helped me to situate that story in a wider human experience. This interest led me to complete a Master of Science in Bioethics in 2016. While there are many ways to think about the role of bioethics in modern healthcare, I adopt a more critical take and frequently delve into critical bioethics literature as a way to analyze and make sense of healthcare activities and structures.

I routinely present on, among other things, the importance of critical thinking in clinical practice. As part of a series of lectures, I was asked to comment on this "new" trend of engaging patients in organizational practices. It seemed at the time a passing topic – something to consider for a short while, then move on. However, it's become increasingly difficult to extract myself from the conversation, not only because the topic itself is fascinating but also because of the role I play in the wider discourse: I am the ultimate engaged patient. Patients like me – articulate, productive, well respected, presentable – are in high demand as presenters and advisers. Although these engagements can produce arguably positive outcomes, the overall use of patients to achieve certain organizational agendas can be exploitative, tokenistic, and even demeaning. (The irony is not lost on me that by critiquing patient engagement, and frequently being asked to write and present on it, I fulfill the very function I aim to dismantle.)

Despite, or perhaps because of, my experiences and training, unlike Paula, I cannot say that I'm interested in making healthcare "better." Rather, I'm interested in understanding and revealing underexplored dynamics and conditions – weighty concepts such as populism, consumerism, and governmentality make their way into my work – even as more and more patients and organizations rally behind formalized patient engagement programs. Whether in writing or in presentations, I resist invitations to advise organizations and practitioners on how to improve their programs. This task is best left to quality, risk, and communications professionals. My work with Paula on this particular project is no different. Here, we do not focus on solutions. Instead, as we consider the intersections of compassionate care, technology, and patient engagement, I take a rare moment to allow myself to consider possibilities. To imagine.

It is from these standpoints that we consider how current – and future – patient engagement practices might have a role to play in creating compassionate care.

CONNECTING CONCEPTS: PRACTICES OF ENGAGEMENT AND PRINCIPLES OF COMPASSION

Patient engagement programs can themselves be understood as a kind of technology. Just as the user interface of an app on a phone renders invisible all of the coding decisions and programs that operate in the background, patient engagement activities can obscure the underlying concepts that animate them. To understand any complex social process, there are layers of assumptions, concepts, and traditions to be unpacked. In socially oriented programs like patient engagement, the concepts are not from fields like computer science or engineering. They derive from the social sciences, health policy, critical theory, political science, organizational studies, and the humanities. These programs pull together many big ideas about how we want to *be* in healthcare, as patients and providers. More broadly, they may reflect who we want to be as a society. Ideas this substantial are bound to get conceptually messy.

In writing this chapter, we needed to wrestle with how we think about patient engagement programs and how we relate those concepts to constructs of compassion. Because compassion is typically defined as a response to suffering, this led us to wonder about the meaning of suffering. But we could not stop in this heavy conceptual territory.

We also needed to connect all of these ideas back to the future imaginary and wonder: Is there a role for patient engagement practices in preserving the centrality of compassion in an increasingly technological landscape?

Practices of Patient Engagement

By practices we mean the things people do to translate their ideas about patient engagement (e.g., what they hope it will achieve, for whom) into tangible activities. In another sense, practices are the enactments or performances of patient engagement: the things you can see and do. These tangible activities create and rely upon all kinds of physical realities. There are forms to create and complete, orientation materials to develop, people to invite, rooms to book, food to order, funds to be reimbursed, agendas to be set, meeting minutes to be recorded, schedules to be aligned, transportation to be arranged. How those activities are created, coordinated, and displayed suggest different purposes for and assumptions about patient engagement.

We will map out three broad categories of patient engagement practices. The first is concerned with specific outputs and outcomes as defined by organizations. We call this an *instrumentalist approach*. The second is concerned with the rights of patients to influence healthcare and healthcare organizations. This we have labelled a *democratic approach*. Finally, there is an approach concerned with developing humanistic understandings of illness and suffering from those who have been, or currently are, ill. This final approach is less well known in the world of patient engagement, but has a long history in the humanities. We call this a *narrative approach*. We should acknowledge here that although we've delineated clearly defined groupings, some practices or activities may fall into more than one category. At least, it is not always obvious which group a practice may belong in. We will come back to these practices and how each might participate in imagining the future of healthcare. But if we want to anchor that future in compassion, we first need to understand what compassion means.

Unpacking Compassion

In academic literature – and in the definition primarily set out in this book – compassion has two core elements. First, compassion requires the recognition of another's suffering. Second, compassion involves a desire toward action to relieve that suffering (Goetz, Keltner, and Simon-Thomas 2010). This is an action-oriented definition of compassion, where *compassion is a response to suffering*. This definition creates a particular conceptual relationship, where there is an antecedent (something that causes suffering), a stimulus (a display of suffering), and some kind of response (a compassionate act). This definition creates useful conceptual precision, separating compassion from other human emotions such as love, sympathy, and empathy. And yet, this definition introduces certain questions.

First, how should we separate concepts of pain and concepts of suffering? Pain is primarily understood as physical and/or mental distress caused by illness and injury. Suffering, by contrast, is not limited to the experience of the body, but may manifest as grief, regret, fear of death or disability, reduction or loss of physical functioning, change in social status or relations, or a host of other complex emotions (Cassell 1982). Pain and suffering can each exist independently; one can have pain without suffering, and vice versa. Arguably, healthcare organizations have many tools available to address pain. Indeed, much of medical science is geared toward treatment and remediation of pain, as well as the prevention or cure of conditions that have life-limiting potential. However, suffering often constitutes something far more than what medical treatment of disease can address.

Second, what forms of suffering are recognized, by whom? The definition of compassion as a response to suffering is based on a premise that one person's suffering is recognizable to another. Given that suffering is complex, deeply personal, and entrenched in social and cultural expectations of how one ought to act (Ellis, Cobb, et al. 2015), a healthcare provider may not always notice suffering in ways that are accurate, consistent, and sensitive. Herein lies a challenge to the definition of compassion. The recognition of suffering is not an entirely cognitive act. Instead, these acts of noticing are also based on cultural norms. Acts of noticing – and moments of not noticing – may also be influenced by implicit bias. If we are going to understand compassionate healthcare as a response to suffering, we need to contend with the ways compassion may be framed as (an unverified and unverifiable) "diagnosis" of suffering based on many (often implicit) judgments by a healthcare practitioner.

The definition of compassion as a response to suffering has some utility. It offers conceptual precision that social psychologists need to discern – and attempt to measure – compassion as distinct from other human emotions. But this definition of compassion does not entirely capture the essence of what we have each heard through our various travels in the world of patient engagement. It does not entirely capture the essence of what we think people mean when they talk about compassion in healthcare. In everyday terms, compassion is more likely thought of as a proactive and heartfelt recognition of shared humanity – which may not be prompted exclusively by recognition of suffering, but by witnessing of relatable vulnerability. A moment of kindness, a shared laugh, a physical gesture. A human connection.

The importance of this broader approach to compassion is illustrated by Dr Donald Berwick (2009) in his article "What 'Patient-Centred' Should Mean: Confessions of an Extremist." Berwick identifies the current risks of healthcare, the harms inflicted and the suffering experienced through various errors, lapses in coordination, and missed opportunities to ensure patient safety during high-risk moments. However, it is not this kind of avoidable harm and the associated suffering that worries him: "Errors and unreliability are not the main reasons that I fear the inevitable day on which I will become a patient. For, in fighting them, I am aligned with the good hearts and fine skills of my technical caregivers, and I can use my own wit to stand guard against them" (Berwick 2009, w563). Perhaps Berwick's knowledge as a physician protects him from worrying about avoidable harm of these kinds. Yet, despite all that he knows about the prevalence of errors in healthcare, it is the threat to his personal identity and sense of humanity that he fears most:

> What chills my bones is the indignity. It is the loss of influence on what happens to me. It is the image of myself in a hospital gown, homogenized, anonymized, powerless, no longer myself … to be made helpless before my time, to be made ignorant when I want to know, to be made to sit when I wish to stand, to be alone when I need to hold my wife's hand, to eat what I do not wish to eat, to be named what I do not wish to be named, to be told when I wish to be asked, to be awoken when I wish to sleep. (Berwick 2009, w564)

In this framing, suffering is caused by the loss of opportunity to be seen the way one wants to be seen. The various indignities that threaten our sense of self – the experiences of healthcare that are perceived as disempowering, dehumanizing, and devaluing (Coyle 1999) – are antithetical to compassionate care. This then suggests that moments of recognition, where personal identities are recognized and where agency is respected, can themselves be acts of compassion. As opposed to the reactive definition of compassion as a response to suffering, we call this proactive orientation *compassion as recognition*. If we locate compassion within moments of recognition, we shift our attention away from compassion as a response to suffering and instead approach compassion as a commitment to shared experiences of humanity.

These moments of recognition do not presume the suffering of another. Their absence, however, may certainly incite suffering. This approach to compassionate care requires humble attention to the ways we might, despite our best intentions, perpetuate the kinds of affronts that Dr Berwick describes, where patients feel unheard, unseen, and unrecognized, particularly in moments of vulnerability.

In considering the dynamics of recognition, we would be remiss in not also exploring the politics of recognition. As we have already alluded, not all experiences of suffering are equally recognized and valued. We have considered compassion as a response and compassion as recognition. Now, we consider a final conception of compassion – one that demands response and recognition on a broader scale. This form of compassion addresses persistent and widespread causes of suffering, including systemic racism, structural violence, poverty, and social isolation. As Paton and colleagues elaborate in chapter 3 of this book, concepts of social justice cannot be untangled from concepts of compassion. Is it meaningful to say that the healthcare system is striving toward compassionate care, if such striving is not equitably distributed? If we have not achieved compassion for all, have we achieved compassion at all? We add another definition of compassion to our conceptual tool kit: *compassion as social justice*.

We have described three distinct ways of understanding compassion. Each one aligns broadly with a different approach to patient engagement. An understanding of compassion as action aligns with an *instrumentalist* approach. An understanding of compassion as social justice aligns with a *democratic* approach. An understanding of compassion as recognition aligns with a *narrative* approach. In practice, these three approaches to patient engagement are often combined, sometimes confused. However, they all have different implications for the future of compassion in healthcare work.

MAPPING CURRENT PRACTICES
OF PATIENT ENGAGEMENT

Instrumentalist Approaches

In instrumentalist approaches to patient engagement, the purposes of patient engagement are relatively straightforward. At least, it is easy to interpret these aims as straightforward. In this framing, patients are depicted as having access to important and unique knowledge that must be extracted and used to achieve the shared aim of improving healthcare. For example, patients experience transitions between elements of the healthcare system and are therefore well positioned to notice the gaps in care that are invisible to those providers who do not venture from their own sphere. Further, it is often only patients who witness disconnects between espoused practices of professionals and what actually happens in the intimacies of patient care. In this way, patients can act as important process informants (Rowland, McMillan, et al. 2018), supplying information and insight back to the organization about how care practices are actually experienced by patients. In this framing, patient engagement serves as an important means to an even more important end: improved patient care.

The rationales used to describe these kinds of patient engagement programs should be familiar to managers and product developers in other industries, where many similar concepts and tools are put to use. Satisfaction surveys, focus groups, process mapping exercises, and quality improvement events proliferate in this space, as does an accompanying "patient involvement industry" complete with tool kits, guidebooks, and endorsements for best practices of engagement. It is entirely possible to imagine a future where AI algorithms collate patient satisfaction scores, complaints, and preferences to predict what kinds of services – and healthcare providers – patients would most likely value.

There is a growing enthusiasm and momentum for this kind of patient engagement, even as some critical scholars raise potentially troubling questions about the philosophical underpinnings of all this activity and the associated questions about power, representation, and benefit. It is in this arena of patient engagement where much activity seems to be blossoming and flourishing. There is also effort to demonstrate the impact of these patient engagement activities as tools to create quality improvement (Bergerum, Thor, et al. 2019).

These approaches to patient engagement – which very much reflect customer-oriented approaches in other industries – may be well suited to enacting certain kinds of compassion, particularly compassion as a response to suffering. As we know from patient complaints, media reports, and continued prevalence of safety concerns, there are times when the people, practices, and places of healthcare actually contribute to patient suffering. Examples include failing to anticipate or treat pain, providing insufficient protection from hospital-acquired infections, creating unnecessary waits, and showing lack of civility or respect toward patients, family members, and other team members (Mylod and Lee 2013). This instrumentalist approach to patient engagement may be compatible with addressing – and preventing – the suffering that comes from harm created by mistakes, by incivility, or by the institutionalized practices that have become entrenched in healthcare despite their deleterious effects.

However, part of what we want to put forward in this chapter is the proposition that each form of patient engagement, while potentially useful for some manifestations of compassionate care, may create unintended blind spots for other forms of compassionate care. There is a risk that patient engagement practices so strongly tilted toward customer-service logics might miss, or even interfere with, other understandings of compassion.

One critique already directed toward patient engagement practices is that they lack diversity. In the field of patient engagement, there is a rumble of concern that current engagement programs may be primarily occupied by patients who are more privileged, more articulate, more powerful. Here there is a potential disconnect. Those who are the most likely to experience the effects of healthcare harm may be the least likely to be heard in formal patient engagement programs. The patients who participate, regardless of their motivations, may or may not be aware of other patients' life experiences and the various ways in which they have encountered harm and suffering. Thus, one standing critique is rooted in a worry that these programs may inadvertently continue to create processes and practices that benefit only the most privileged.

Often, patient engagement practitioners seek to address this concern by endeavouring to recruit the "hard to reach." Yet, sociologist Ruha Benjamin (2013) suggests that trying to address social justice concerns through more and more recruitment of patients is not likely to ease the various tensions that underpin lack of engagement. Perhaps the problem is not lack of knowledge or time or access to these institutionally sponsored programs. Perhaps it is lack of trust. If a group of people has already experienced systematic marginalization by healthcare practices and organizations, those people are not likely to trust an organizationally sponsored patient engagement program, no matter how extensively recruitment is advertised. Further, simply transposing the same logics of engagement into electronic platforms will not solve the foundational problem of trust, even if the digital forums increase the program's reach. Thus, there is a need to look to other practices of patient engagement that are sensitized to questions of power, voice, and a rights-based approach to shaping the future of healthcare.

Democratic Approaches

Another arena of patient engagement takes on a democratic tone. Beyond using patients' unique knowledge as a resource for improving healthcare services, these practices position patient engagement as a right. In countries where health and healthcare are valued as a social good, there is an accompanying imperative for patients as citizens, taxpayers, and relevant stakeholders to exercise their right to influence healthcare. The distinction between an instrumentalist and a democratic orientation is subtle but important. Consider an instrumentalist way of thinking taken to its logical extreme. According to this logic, if patients are engaged thoroughly and comprehensively, the resultant designs will be well informed and well grounded in patients' needs. A consumerist logic would pursue specific goals that, once achieved, serve as a natural end point for patient engagement. Such an end point would be reached when our healthcare systems met their aspired ideal. Some might argue that AI strategies could reach this ideal state much more quickly than the long, cumbersome process of engaging with people. If Google can predict my shopping preferences based on my digital traces, surely there is a comparable and equally powerful possibility of collating and predicting patients' care preferences.

Now, contrast this to a democratic understanding. There is no end point to a democratic process. The process itself is foundational to the goal. While meaningful change and positive impacts are surely aspired to, there is no point where all parties will agree: "We have reached our aims. We can stop with the democratic process now and go back to the way things were." So, while the *techniques* of patient engagement might look similar, the understanding of value and the relationships of responsibility are quite different in democratic as compared to instrumentalist rationales for patient engagement. The democratic and instrumentalist approaches have different logics, grow from different historical roots, and suggest different futures for engagement. As a result, they have different possibilities for their relationship to compassionate care.

Democratic rationales may have the capacity to address the social justice concerns we raised. Thus, these approaches may be well suited to address compassion as social justice. Here, patient engagement programs anchored in more democratic rationales may eschew techniques better suited for market research and instead engage with strategies such as deliberative dialogue. In this context, deliberation refers to the act of carefully considering different points of view and coming to a reasoned decision. With roots in concepts of democracy, the underlying premise is that diverse groups engaging in genuine listening, understanding, and potentially persuasion will ultimately lead to better, more reasoned, and public-spirited decisions (Abelson, Forest, et al. 2003).

However, the value of democracy registers on a different kind of scale, with an emphasis on process and participation. Therefore, programs would be evaluated in very different ways. Here, the aim is to create health systems responsive to the concerns of those that they are meant to serve. Patient engagement practices exclusively based on democratic rationales may fall short of addressing the micro-practices of healthcare that can lead to harm. As discussed, these might be better addressed through instrumentalist approaches and strategies of quality improvement. However, there is yet another arena of compassion that is still potentially missed, even if democratic and instrumentalist practices complement one another. We now turn our attention to compassion as recognition.

Narrative Approaches

While patient engagement programs grounded in instrumentalist rationales favour strategic forms of communication ("What are we to do?"), narrative approaches favour dialogic communication. Dialogue refers to a particular way of communicating that is about entering a thought process and collectively changing how that process occurs (Bohm 1996). It is a form of inquiry, of thinking and reflecting together (Issacs 1999). As an approach, dialogic communication opens the possibility of truly engaging with another, of other voices shaping our own voice, allowing ourselves to be potentially destabilized, to see ourselves differently (Frank 2004). In this way, dialogic communication creates the space and the conditions that allow for mutual explorations of how we are to *be*. Engaging with patient narratives provides the opportunity to recognize – and be influenced by – the lifeworld of someone who has experienced illness, who has suffered. As sociologist Arthur Frank (2013, 145) describes, "By conceiving suffering as pedagogy, agency is restored to ill people; testimony is given equal place alongside professional expertise." In this way, narrative practices of patient engagement are concerned with transformative learning, identity development, and reflexivity (Hawthornthwaite, Roebotham, et al. 2018).

Such approaches raise and confront questions of how to be human, how to recognize each other in moments of illness, even (and especially) when suffering cannot be avoided or resolved. There is no hiding from the twinned paths of pain and longevity when life-saving treatments include surgeries, risk-laden medications, or other such interventions. Here, new metaphors of compassion are introduced: compassion as witnessing, as negotiating deep and unresolvable tensions, as acknowledging difference, as maintaining humility. Compassion as mutual human generosity, exploring questions of health, illness, and how to live (Frank 2004). These metaphors of compassion stand in contrast to our more commonly held understandings of compassion as action. Narrative approaches to patient engagement may be well suited to fostering *compassion as recognition*, where learning from pedagogies of suffering helps us be more present, more human, to see one another (and ourselves) more clearly in these moments of care.

However, the current momentum around patient engagement certainly seems to favour action-oriented, problem-focused strategies. It is difficult to demonstrate impact of narrative approaches, at least in the way the healthcare system tends to think about impact along predefined and measurable parameters. Further, the emphasis on power and power-sharing as a defining feature of patient engagement does not lend itself to demonstrating the value of narrative approaches. There is a risk that these approaches may be dismissed as "just storytelling" and "tokenistic." Even more troublesome, there is a worry that these stories of illness could be co-opted, put into service of organizational imperatives, participating in incremental improvements of existing systems and more "business as usual."

And yet, there is something important about the notion of pedagogies of suffering. These approaches create space to learn from patients in narrative ways, without being entirely sure how that learning can be translated into material effects. This may involve learning (and relearning) how to be compassionate as bad news is delivered, as patients and families grapple with difficult decisions, as individuals come to grips with irrevocably changed futures. This framing of compassion allows us to consider moral moments invoked in the presence of suffering that cannot be resolved within the domains of biomedicine. As we move into a future with more and more emphasis on technology, this capacity may become even more important. Not everything is amenable to fixing; some forms of suffering cannot be mitigated by healthcare providers. And yet, healthcare providers acting in the liminal spaces of life and death often find themselves in proximity to this kind of suffering. The instabilities, threats, and suffering that are part of life – and death – cannot be managed through technology alone (Cribb 2017). Other forms of response are needed. Any future that proposes to offer both health and care must be capable of this wide repertoire. Any forms of patient engagement that seek to enable compassionate care must also make room for these humanistic understandings of illness, suffering, and humanity.

WHERE WE ARE NOW

Patient engagement programs often cite compassionate care among their aims. In this chapter, we have explored the meaning of compassion in order to consider how this ideal might be enabled and constrained by different approaches to patient engagement. This took us into some conceptual territory that is relatively underexplored in the patient engagement literature, perhaps surprisingly so. We explored alternate conceptualizations of compassion, building upon the most widely accepted notion of *compassion as a response to suffering* to introduce *compassion as recognition* and to hold space for *compassion as social justice*. If compassion is an ideal of care, and we are enrolling patients to help shape or improve care, we should be curious about how programs of patient engagement support and influence our understanding of compassion.

What we find are patient engagement programs that tend to be aligned with action-oriented ideals of compassion. They pursue actions that produce measurable solutions to visible problems as they are defined by the healthcare organization. The manner in which patients are involved could be described as orderly and well managed, fitting neatly into corporate and organizational culture with minimal risk of disruption. This instrumentalist approach allows certain solutions, particularly solutions aligned with logics of quality improvement. We certainly need to continue to improve processes and practices that are currently inefficient, uncoordinated, and even overtly unsafe. However, we must also be willing to recognize that when patient engagement programs operationalize this ideal of compassion or limit compassion to the realm of "measurable outcomes," the healthcare organizations themselves maintain control over patients' experiences and the possible definitions of the problems at hand. Controlling the agenda is one of the most effective displays of organizational power (Lukes 2005), no matter how well-intentioned that agenda-setting might be. These instrumentally oriented programs necessarily shift focus away from exploring other equally pressing questions.

We also tend to find patient engagement programs that combine (and sometimes confuse) various approaches to patient engagement. Such blurring can add to a sense of incoherence and internal conflict within various patient programs, a dilemma that vexes program planners, patients, and researchers. For example, a patient may be invited to "tell their story" but feel constrained by organizational norms to only tell a particular kind of story, for a particular kind of instrumental purpose, in a particular way. They may wish to express their rights as a citizen but find the agendas of meetings already set, decisions already made, and their role limited to that of a savvy consumer. Given how the consumerist paths of patient engagement are positioned as so promising, enticing, and tangible, these instrumentalist ways of doing patient engagement might overshadow other ways of learning that are less concrete, less measurable, and less obviously tied to constructs such as "impact." As such, even the more democratic or narrative patient engagement programs may get pressed into service as quality improvement interventions.

WHERE WE MIGHT GO

If we are willing to accept that compassion encompasses multiple meanings and concepts – compassion as response to suffering, as recognition, as social justice – and we aim for patient engagement programs to contribute to this vision of compassionate care, then we need to take a clear-eyed look at how practices of patient engagement may advance some elements of compassion while potentially disrupting or distracting from others.

We worry that the more instrumental ways of understanding patient engagement will only continue to grow as they interface with the various technological advances that will define the future of healthcare. After all, the logics of consumerism, customer service, and product development that occupy instrumentalist frames of patient engagement are a natural fit with the growing industry of healthcare products and services. As patient engagement practices continue to tilt toward the strategic, we wonder what will be lost. Perhaps we will find ourselves triumphant in vanquishing avoidable suffering as part of the healthcare experience; hopefully, for all. And yet, in the process, we might lose sight of our capacity to be present in the face of suffering that is not resolvable through biomedical means. In listening to patients' stories selectively and using them for predefined purposes we may fail to see and learn from patients on their own terms. In the rush to prevent and resolve some forms of suffering, we may inadvertently create others.

If patient engagement practices seek to expand our collective capacity for compassion, we must be ever mindful of the ways in which we are pulled, perhaps inevitably, toward the technocratic, instrumentalized forms of patient engagement outlined in this chapter. This instrumental and incremental approach may limit the ways we can respond to the variable needs of patient populations as we continue to face new challenges as healthcare – and society – change. To that end, a fundamental question lingers, which is far bigger in scope than we have allowed ourselves to ask so far: Is it even possible for a non-technocratic patient engagement intervention to be properly *imagined*, let alone implemented, by those immersed in a technocratic culture? Can patient engagement programs – initiated, sustained, and nurtured by healthcare institutions – be anything but instrumental?

While we feel it is a useful exercise to challenge constructed boundaries of our own making, we also concede that the pull of the consumerist framing is very strong. So we recognize it may come to pass that we cannot somehow "engage" our way out of this instrumental framing or simply rethink patient engagement into something less instrumental. If there is hope for compassion in healthcare as a way to address suffering, it may have to come from a place not constructed by the same forces that forged modern healthcare. We may also look to philosophy, to the humanities, to various social movements, or to other patient-led streams of activity that are not bound to the same instrumental and technocratic logics that seem to be nearly inevitable in the growing patient engagement industry. This still positions medicine and healthcare as essential dialogical partners for patients, but it does not allow healthcare professionals to retain sole authorship of how the future of healthcare should unfold.

NOTE

1   We are using the term *patient* as an overarching category to include all those who have experienced healthcare services from the standpoint of receiving care. For ease of writing this chapter, we will include patients, caregivers, and family members within this same category of "patient." This rhetorical choice is consistent with current international trends in the field. However, we recognize the limits of these word choices. A discussion about the challenge of language in patient engagement programs and policies is important to consider and explore but is beyond the scope of this chapter.

3

Care in the Real World: Partial Perspectives on Compassion, Technology, and Equity

Morag Paton, Thirusha Naidu, Lisa Richardson, Arno Kumagai, and Ayelet Kuper

You wake up slowly, as the lights in your suburban Canadian bedroom move gradually from dark to light. Your phone, which is charging on your bedside table, starts playing your favourite song, at first quietly, then louder. You sit up, check the time, and start your day. Your watch shows that you got more REM sleep than you did the night before, which is great because you have a lot of meetings scheduled today and have to be on your toes. You're annoyed, though, because you see that you are still below the average amount of REM sleep for people in your same demographic. You're in the kitchen now, pouring your morning cup of coffee. Then you head out to your car, while your watch silently records every step, every heartbeat, every location. You pay a little extra on your parking app to get a premium spot closer to your office, but once inside, you take the stairs instead of the elevator, so you can tell your doctor that you have actually started exercising five days a week. The walks you have told her you were taking at lunch were, in reality, trips to order takeout, which you ate while browsing on Amazon from your office chair. Life is stressful, there is a lot to do, and your health does not always top your priority list. But you think your watch is helping you change all that.

Health wearables are a rapidly growing segment of the tech economy, purported to increase our knowledge about how our own body functions, improve our sleep patterns, encourage us to exercise, and make us accountable. We can track our heart rate, REM sleep, and stairs climbed. We can track our next period, optimize our workouts, send our location to a loved one, and compare our activities with friends.

The computer whirls. It sees that your sleep improved, and a green check mark appears in a column within your profile page. It can see that your calendar today is busy, so a red *X* appears in the other column. It can recognize your stress levels. Another red *X* appeared when your heart rate spiked while you sat in heavy traffic on your way to the office. Taking the stairs helped a bit, but the device's calculations show that you did not burn off the calories from the meal you ordered online the night before. Another red *X*. It can see that you have been sedentary for most of the day. Red *X*. It runs its daily diagnostic report. Your discount for your life insurance has just changed from 10 per cent to only 5 per cent. Your car insurance rates adjust, recognizing the heavy traffic you're in and the stress you're under, and by the end of the month, you're paying twenty dollars more. Your doctor's office sends you a notification, asking you to schedule an appointment sooner. Your standing online grocery order adds heart-healthy leafy greens and removes the bag of sweet and salty popcorn you enjoy. Your period tracker app notifies your employer that you may be pregnant.

How far off is this scenario exactly? Some of this may feel familiar, some of it more dystopian fiction. Some of it may seem benign and helpful, and some of it may seem invasive and terrifying. Health wearables and mobile health data recorders are being built and deployed to increase access to our own health data. Devices are available that allow us to test our own cortisol levels through home monitors and mobile apps to measure and improve stress levels (see www.inmehealth.com). Apps on our hand-held devices are used as social platforms, enabling women to build self-help groups without the fear of social stigma in their own communities (e.g., www.whatsapp.com). Hand-held and wearable devices can identify glaucoma, augment eyesight to detect obstacles, monitor disease, and reduce the need for people to travel to urban centres for testing. Conceivably, wearable devices can allow for a health worker speaking one language to easily communicate with a sick patient who speaks another. As all of this

Technology

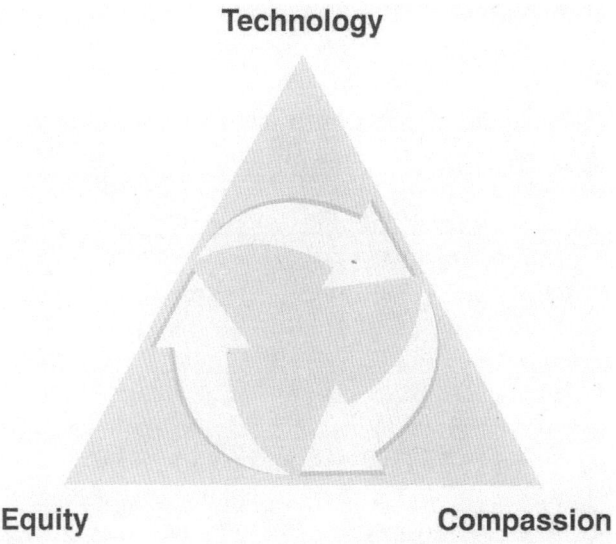

Equity   **Compassion**

Figure 3.1 Compassion, equity, and technology triangle

is going on, technology corporations are partnering with health insurance companies, genetic testing results are being shared with corporate and legal entities, and privacy breaches are releasing data onto the web.

Many technological advances purport to offer us information, choice, and freedom. They may allow physicians to provide compassionate, patient-centred care focused on the patient's personal needs and contexts. Well-intentioned technologies offer hope in cases where there may have once been little. The promise of technology, however, is offset by risks and unintended consequences that operate on a larger scale and demand our close attention.

In this chapter, we trouble current discussions about the relationship between technology and compassion, arguing there is a third entity that exists in tension with both: equity (figure 3.1). We argue that equity must be considered in any discussion of the ways in which technology will impact the possibilities for compassionate care. Without careful attention to equity, we cannot adequately take stock of emerging technologies and their effects.

For example, how might wearables that track location affect groups of people who need ID cards to live on their ancestral lands, people who may be stopped by the police because of the colour of their skin and the neighbourhood in which they are walking, or people who were once rounded up and sent to concentration camps with the help of technologies that allowed them to be counted, tracked, and exterminated? What influence might wearables have on employees who continue lifestyles that increase the insurance costs of their employers? How might a period tracking app influence a newly pregnant, under-resourced, and scared teenage girl if she lives in a state that is advancing anti-abortion legislation? What influence might wearables have in places where people are more concerned about access to clean water, housing, or food than their car insurance premiums or hitting their 10,000 steps a day?

As authors of this chapter, we differ in our geographical settings and in our histories. We differ in our training, affiliations, professions, and experiences. We hold varied perspectives and different kinds of power and influence. We share the conviction that compassion requires equity. We argue in this chapter that without equity, compassionate care is the purview of the privileged minority who own, control, and/or benefit from the technology. While some technologies may promise to democratize care, inequities still exist, and these may not be erased (and may indeed be heightened) through technology.

We frame this chapter in four sections. First, we discuss compassion. We argue that the meaning of compassion must be considered from multiple perspectives, not imposed by those empowered to define suffering and provide care. Second, we discuss technology. Building on Ursula Franklin's concept of the real world of technology, we suggest that we should ask not what technologies are but what they are doing. Third, we introduce the concept of equity, applying it to the context of women's health and HIV/AIDS. Finally, we discuss reflective practice as a way to enhance compassionate and equitable care.

ON COMPASSION

Showing compassion is often considered akin to being a good person, and receiving compassionate care is analogous to being treated well. *The Oxford Handbook of Compassion Science* defines compassion as "a state of concern for the suffering or unmet need of another, coupled with a desire to alleviate that suffering" (Goetz and Simon-Thomas 2017). We argue that this definition has been conceived and applied within healthcare primarily by privileged groups working within a Western context. We consider the limits of this definition, exploring different perspectives about what compassionate care is, what it may look like, and how to achieve it.

A single definition of compassion (such as the one above) may be a problematic imposition in a world view and context different from that of the white female American authors of that handbook. A singular definition of compassion has been applied in narrow and culturally specific ways. Instead, how might compassion need to be conceptualized and operationalized differently to provide compassionate, culturally conscious care in other contexts? In the countries where the authors of this chapter live, how might the Indigenous peoples of Canada and South Africa envision and operationalize compassion as settlers continue to occupy their ancestral lands?

Different cultures and individuals have different constructions of what compassion and compassionate care may mean. Defining compassion as a relationship between one individual and another may not be congruent with world views that embrace the well-being of a community over the well-being of any one individual within it. We carry diverse understandings of suffering and compassion, shaped by our unique experiences, knowledge, and upbringing. Critically examining the idea of compassion means we need to be ready to consider different perspectives of what that may look like and how to achieve it.

PARTIAL PERSPECTIVES ON COMPASSION

The different ways in which we construct compassion and compassionate care stem from our different perspectives. In this section, we look to writers who have provided insight into the nature of perspectives as they relate to technologies and to our understanding of the world. In so doing, we challenge assumptions about what compassion means and what compassionate care could look like.

Some writers challenge the very nature of science (Haraway 1988; Harding 1992). In the development of Western science after the Enlightenment, science had been regarded as something that was continually improving our world. Scientists strived to unravel the mysteries of the universe, seeking out truth and answers to their unsolved questions. They believed the answers were out there and only needed to be found. Western science was posited as neutral, rational, and innocent (Bristow 2011). Science was uncontested and believed to be advancing us all toward a better future.

These "truths" and the privilege afforded to Western science have continuously been challenged within the Global South. In one example, Boaventura de Sousa Santos, a Portuguese sociologist who conducted extensive field work in Brazil, raises these issues in his book *Another Knowledge Is Possible: Beyond Northern Epistemologies* (2008). He directly critiques the "hegemonic conception of modern scientific knowledge" (de Sousa Santos 2008, xxviii), the suppression of Indigenous knowledges through colonization, and the creation of the "other" as a manufactured inferior being. Similar concepts can be seen in the work of Edward Said, who was born in British-ruled Palestine in the 1930s to a Palestinian mother and an American father. *Orientalism* (Said 1979) exposes how colonial forces manufactured differences between those in the Global North and those in the Global South in order to create an "alien" that needed to be rescued and tamed. Said's work argues that colonialism was not just a way of spreading one civilization but also a way of destroying others. Argentinian scholar Walter Mignolo (Mignolo and Walsh 2018) speaks of the totalizing effects of Eurocentrism, arguing for pluralist voices and the constitution and reconstitution of a "decolonial" way of thinking. Other examples from India, Canada, and South Africa (Dei and Johal 2005; Ndofirepi and Gwaravanda 2018; Sardar 1988; Spivak 1994) show that this is indeed a well-established global phenomenon.

In the Global North, Haraway (1988) asserts that science is neither neutral nor innocent, but instead science (and therefore the way we see the world) is affected by power. What can be known as "true" or "scientific" can be modified depending on context, power, or privilege. People who hold power can assert the "science" they feel would best serve their own interests. People who hold less power may find this more difficult. For Haraway (1988, 1991), there is no such thing as a universal truth or objective knowledge. Instead, there are multiple truths and multiple types of knowledge that emerge from the various perspectives and identities of those who are creating this knowledge. If history has been written by the victor, then science has been constructed by the powerful.

Where there are multiple truths and types of knowledge, there is no universal truth or truly objective knowledge. Instead, our perspectives are *partial, subjective, and context dependent*, and these views are shaped and coloured by what we have learned through our upbringing, our histories, and our lived experiences. No individual can ever see the full perspective. No individual can ever grasp the full "truth." Instead, our perspectives are always filtered through our own subjectivities; through our way of seeing, thinking, or learning about the world. Yet often it is the people in power who declare their knowledge to be true or another's knowledge to be false. There are no "gold standards" in compassionate care, because constructing one would entail wielding power over others' experiences. As Tassone and colleagues argue in chapter 6 of this book, a sustainable, compassionate environment needs leadership that is authentic, self-aware, and generative. And within this authentic self-awareness, those who have the privilege to hold power at any given moment need to recognize that their perspectives, too, are partial – incomplete and always evolving.

Coupled with this dynamic of partial perspectives and power, our own identities change over time. They develop through and are modified by our interactions with family, community, and others. Technology has changed the way people interact with each other: people can build relationships online, they can text instead of talk, and can make lasting friendships with people they'll never even meet. Whereas once people may have interacted primarily with those in their own village or town or school, technology allows us to reach well beyond those geographic limitations. One's identity with a group may no longer be based on common social constructions such as race and gender. Our identities need not be rooted in our hometowns, our families, or the expectations that we grew up with. Instead, increasing technology may allow us to reconstruct our identities through our relationships and affinities with others. We can become something else, learn something different, and modify the learned behaviours passed down to us from our families, teachers, and peers. Not only are our perspectives partial but also our identities can change over time. What we once thought was "fixed" is instead something that is "floating."

Those who practice in healthcare may identify themselves as providers of compassionate care. Those who hold power in healthcare may enact strategies they also believe are compassionate. But within this context, our learned behaviours and partial perspectives may actually shield us from what is going on. Practices that may have seemed compassionate to a healthcare professional, for example, may appear quite different when that same professional becomes a patient themselves. Sometimes "care" is not compassionate. What one person may see as compassionate may actually seem cruel to another.

One of this chapter's authors spent the first two weeks of her life away from her parents, having been airlifted to another hospital shortly after her birth. To the doctors and advisers this was seen as compassionate, ensuring that she received the care she needed. To the mother who was left behind and placed in a recovery ward full of newborns nestled next to their own mothers, this was seen as necessary but cruel. If we are ever to achieve compassionate care for each individual, we need to start asking what compassion means from multiple points of view. As technology allows our identities to shift and our partial perspectives to expand, one can hope that our understandings of what compassion means, or what compassionate care looks like or feels like, can also expand. Received definitions of compassion (or equity) will need to be contested. Non-dominant perspectives will need to be given room to challenge any seemingly simple, taken-for-granted definition. Leaders and other people in positions of authority will need to not only recognize the perspectives of others but also support and promote others with these perspectives so that system-level change can occur.

Changes can be supported through institutional shifts in policy and the expansion of consultation processes to promote perspectives not traditionally considered. System-level changes can be supported through critical reflection. One needs to recognize that any given definition of compassion or expression of compassionate care is socially situated, subjective, manifested individually, and filtered through different social locations, privileges, and relative access to resources (Harding 1992). A watch that tracks your steps and encourages you to get moving may be seen by some as a beneficial fitness enabler but a total invasion of privacy to others. Instead of declaring that only one of these perspectives is "true," those who design, market, or use these technologies need to critically reflect on why they think this technology is useful and consider it from another perspective as well. Being critically reflective, interrogating our own "truths," and recognizing our own partial perspectives creates space for the addition of others: our individual filter broadens.

Linda Tuhiwai Smith (1999) offers a different way to broaden perspectives – one resting within the cultural, historical, and epistemological traditions of her own Maori culture. She advocates for collaborative, community-based inquiry that underpins movements for social change. Smith argues for respectful and enabling processes where different perspectives from different historical and cultural traditions can work together. Collaborative, community-based inquiry is emancipatory and inclusive, centred around and led by the people it would most affect. For Smith (1999), change needs to be collaborative and based within the communities that it will serve. Without this important first step, then the dominant "truth" will always lead.

If health leaders want to understand how to enact compassionate care, they need to understand that their own perspectives are partial; interrogate their advantages; seek out, value, and centre perspectives that are not their own; and, if necessary, remove themselves entirely from the centre of the discussion, allowing others to determine their own definition of compassion, what compassionate care may look like, and how it may be achieved.

How can this approach work in practice? Smith's work offers multiple helpful examples, including several based in strategies to build Indigenous research capacity in the knowledge economy (Smith 1999, 2008). In the changing technology of genomics, for example, she suggests that Indigenous researchers should contextualize the effects of technology within colonialism. This serves two purposes: a form of documentation and a form of resistance to changes that negatively impact Indigenous populations. Smith (1999, 2008) describes contextualizing technology through the perspective of Indigenous peoples and through the lens of colonization as a way of disrupting change and offering an alternative. Can wearable technology be a potential technological solution to increasing access to health monitoring for remotely located Indigenous peoples? Or are wearables simply an extension of the laws that seek to categorize, locate, and control while further distancing Indigenous peoples away from traditional medicine?

As a group of authors, we also need to be reflective and recognize our own privileges. We are all employed in academia in some way, where teaching and learning are part of our everyday work. Our basic needs are met in our respective countries by our salaries and stipends. The knowledge claims we make as a group are indeed situated in the time and places from which they came. The fact that we can even debate the definition of compassion means that we are privileged in our own rights, with the advantage of access to communication technology, support, time, freedom, and a voice. Many individuals challenge notions of compassion every day, but do not have the privileges that we do to have their perspectives read, heard, or acknowledged. At the same time, as a group of individuals, we also have our own identities, histories, and belief systems, each very different from one another, that affect how we see compassion, technology, and equity. While we may seem at times to speak as one voice, there are in fact multiple voices in this chapter, each of us providing a glimpse into our own partial perspectives and identities. As Haraway (1988) ultimately asserts, we need to live with discordance instead of harmony, knowing that knowledge claims from any single source (including this one) need to be questioned and opened up for challenges, debates, and subsequent modification.

A singular definition of compassion is therefore inadequate. Those in power within healthcare, including some of the authors listed in this chapter, enact compassionate care and do so from within their own privileged and dominant perspectives. New and evolving definitions of compassion and compassionate care would be helpful but still ineffective if the continual reinforcement of power contributes to marginalization and supports ongoing structural inequities. As we enact compassionate care, we must consider how these enactments reinforce our own privileged and dominant perspectives. Whose versions of compassion get enacted, and whose versions are excluded from these enactments?

TECHNOLOGIES

Some advocates argue that technology can help re-centre compassionate care, closing the gaps facing vulnerable populations. Telemedicine, for example, has brought expertise to the bedside in some remote Indigenous communities in Canada, minimizing the risks inherent in transporting a patient to a centralized location (Khan, Ndubuka, et al. 2017). We know that mobile health technologies can enable the reach of HIV testing into rural communities and increase adherence and continuity of care (Catalani, Philbrick, et al. 2013; King, Kinvig, et al. 2017). Those in power make compelling arguments that high-end technology is needed for efficient or equitable or even compassionate healthcare (Bhatia and Falk 2018; Canada 2017). These arguments may be wrong.

The introduction of new technologies does not necessarily improve lives. For example, ask a parent of a pre-teen or a teacher in an urban centre in Canada today how they feel about mobile technology, and you will likely hear conflicting opinions about how it enables communication in one way but destroys it in another. Dinner may be on the table, but the kids are still downstairs just finishing up their online game. What about the use of Dr Google? How did we get to the point where you notice a bump on your leg and within two internet searches and four websites, you've diagnosed yourself with a deadly skin disease? What about apps on phones that allow for health reporting in underserviced communities or contact-tracing apps to prevent viral spread? Do they lead to better health outcomes or do they increase surveillance? On the one hand, we can be armed with more information than ever before. On the other hand, we may not know what it means, how to interpret it, or how it's changing how we live.

Franklin (1999) describes technology as a *practice* or as *a way we do things*. In defining technology as a practice in which we engage, Franklin moves the idea out of the realm of computer chips and machines and humanizes technology. Like others have done for Western science, Franklin also rejects the notion that technology is neutral. She recognizes that the introduction of technology changes how humans work and live and how we construct ourselves as social beings.

Franklin divides technology into two categories: holistic technologies and prescriptive technologies. Holistic technologies are controlled by the worker. These technologies emerged largely from craft industries and allow the worker to maintain control over their craft. Examples include carpentry or cooking. The individual worker decides how they use technologies based on their experiences and expertise, and they can shape the work as they go. How we work with prescriptive technologies differs. Instead of maintaining control, control is given up with prescriptive technologies. The worker can no longer shape their own work, and the technologies demand that each worker perform only a single step in a longer chain of required interventions. Assembly-line workers are the most obvious example, but this could extend to many groups who work with routine documentation processes, for example. The worker using prescriptive technologies is guided by instruction rather than experience.

The danger of prescriptive technologies is that they change our practice of work. Instead of reducing inequities by creating jobs and profit, the rise of prescriptive technologies has, in many cases, worsened inequities. Franklin argues that the rampant increase of these prescriptive technologies, which are more easily scaled up and distributed, has led to shifts in power. Relationships between government and people have changed. Now, planning and infrastructure are geared toward accommodating prescriptive technologies, rather than the humans who use them, and this, Franklin states, has created a culture of compliance. This culture means that we are more likely to accept a single way of doing something over what had previously been considered a series of personal choices or options. Passwords now limit our access to certain data, swipe cards now limit our access to certain places, and sophisticated technology now limits our ability to repair things on our own. The culture of compliance means that the introduction of technologies has eliminated options. Whereas, in the past, individuals would use principles and experience to decide between options (*a*), (*b*), or (*c*), technology now eliminates the first two options from us, forcing us to comply with option (*c*) alone. These limits can be a way of managing risk, but they can also remove our ability to make decisions. We are no longer citizens; we are consumers, and as consumers, we engage with technologies in a scripted way. Some of us didn't get to write that script.

Franklin gives the historical example of the sewing machine as a technology that promised freedom but delivered something different. In the nineteenth century, advertisements proclaimed the advent of the sewing machine. They promised women more freedom once they were liberated from the time-consuming task of hand sewing. It was assumed that the same people who had always done the sewing would continue to do so; they would simply do it faster and more easily. However, as the technology became more and more prescriptive and standardized, the act of sewing moved from the home to the factory. From there, it moved from the factory to the sweatshop, with these sweatshops actively exploiting mostly immigrant female workers. Sewing was no longer done in the home but by exploited labour and, increasingly, automation. The prescriptive technology of the sewing machine promised liberation but resulted in inequity.

Liberation has not exactly happened, either, with the introduction of technologies in our modern days. Even deliberate attempts to promote "inclusive innovation" have been mixed as firms in the Global North continue to invest in the Global South, taking advantage of cheap labour costs but not necessarily reinvesting in those communities. Since the global economic crisis in 2008, rapid economic growth in China, Sub-Saharan Africa, and India has been met with an actual decline in the income of the poorest people (Chataway, Hanlin, and Kaplinsky 2014). In the Global North, there is growing concern that one day people may not be able to opt out of wearable technology, their health data being relayed to their employers, healthcare practitioners, and insurers (Montgomery, Chester, and Kopp 2018). Indeed, this is far from liberating.

The social opportunities and costs of new technologies are incalculable. We cannot know what burdens we may be assuming ourselves or passing on to others. We argue for the examination of technology as practices and the awareness that these practices emerge from and construct social structures in particular historical contexts. When there is an opportunity to employ a new technology, we need to understand not only what that technology is or how much it costs, but also how it changes our work. We need to understand how technologies can create or eliminate access to multiple perspectives and, most importantly, what technology does to us and to our communities.

How the introduction and proliferation of AI in healthcare will ultimately change who we are as a people, as health practitioners, as educators, or as patients and families is as yet unknown. We do know we must examine the assumption that AI will improve our health outcomes. It may do so for some of us but not for all of us. The opportunities that AI can bring to healthcare are increasingly promoted by those in power and those who are the nexus of healthcare, the economy, and political will (Bhatia and Falk 2018; Canada 2017). AI-based prediction machines are improving in quality and dropping in price (Agrawal, Gans, and Goldfarb 2018). More and more of us are using wearable technologies. Fitness monitors and smart watches collect data on heart rates and this data is being used to predict and diagnose heart disease. While there is significant concern about the impact of technologies on jobs and professions (R. Susskind and D. Susskind 2015), red flags are also raised to alert us about the impact of AI on the distribution of wages, predicting that there will be winners and losers in the competition from trade with machines. Like the owners of the sewing machine, the owners of AI may be well positioned to gain advantages, while those who are tasked with the production of the machines themselves may not be so well positioned.

One way in which technologies have changed how we do things is through our evolving relationship to time. Franklin (1999) contrasts what she calls the bitsphere, our digital world, with the biosphere, our natural world. Within that world is the sequencing of nature: the turn of the Earth, the pull of the moon, or the rising of the sun. Our relationship to time has developed through this biosphere and we have developed myths, religion, and science to make sense of this. We have developed order, sequence, and correlation, even as we do harm to the biosphere in which we live. In contrast, the bitsphere has no such structure and order. It is asynchronous, fragmented, and timeless. Patterns have changed. People have been displaced by devices and feel socially dislocated. Within the bitsphere we have considerable access to knowledge and data, but our actual understanding of that knowledge is weaker. We assume that access to technology, knowledge, and data will enable and enrich us, but what we need to consider is how that access has changed us. As our work is increasingly dislocated, our ability to work together in teams may be harmed. As our work is increasingly depersonalized, perhaps our ability to work compassionately may be diminished. As our work is increasingly fragmented and placed on the global marketplace, perhaps our ability to work toward improved living conditions for everyone is at risk.

History shows that groups who are structurally marginalized may suffer more from technological change purported to improve human health. Cells from Henrietta Lacks, a farmer, parent, and Black woman in 1950s America, were taken without her consent and used in genomic research. HeLa cells continue to be used unethically. Her entire genomic sequence was published online without the consent of her genetic descendants (Skloot 2010, 2013). Vaccine trials in developing countries also demonstrate how the structurally marginalized may suffer due to changes in knowledge and technology. Lack of proper informed consent techniques has resulted in people who live in the most under-resourced places being unethically recruited into vaccine trials (Panagiotou, Katsaragakis, et al. 2009). The bitsphere continues to collide with these important ethical issues. There may well be a risk of introducing AI to the profession of medicine, but there will also be significant economic and social implications to society.

There are many more examples that demonstrate this. In the "Cyborg Manifesto," Haraway (1991) asserts that the technology continuously gazing down at us with a "view from above" provides us with a false vision which separates humans from reality. Instead she advocates for an embodied "view from below," rooted in our experiences and embodied opinions. Critical scholars increasingly are raising their concerns about the introduction of new technologies, what they mean, who controls them, and how they will change us. Ruha Benjamin, a sociologist at Princeton University, offers multiple critiques of the discriminatory nature of science and technology through her works. In one of her books, *People's Science*, she grapples with the history of stem cell research and the predatory nature of this research on marginalized communities (Benjamin 2013). In another of which she is editor, *Captivating Technology*, she wraps a series of chapters about discriminatory design around an argument that calls for and exemplifies the bridging of science and technology studies with critical race studies (Benjamin 2019). In *Algorithms of Oppression*,

Noble (2018) argues, for example, that search engines are imbued with practices that discriminate against Black women in particular. If whiteness is privileged in our search engines according to Noble, then it would stand to reason that whiteness is equally as privileged in the algorithms that purport to deliver healthcare. If the view from above is discriminatory and predatory, and if our healthcare technology is built upon this view, then we need to attend instead to the views from below, full of partial perspectives, in order to give or receive truly compassionate care.

Complacency is untenable. As political, economic, and healthcare leaders look to technologies to solve some of the gaps in our systems, advocates for equity and compassionate care need to challenge them to articulate what the purposes of those technologies are, who stands to gain from their introduction, and who stands to lose (Benjamin 2013). Reflection and meaningful community consultation would certainly propel these conversations forward. Once identified, stakeholders need to ask if the consequences are worthwhile because, as Franklin (1999) and many others assert, the introduction of technology is not neutral, but changes how we work, who we are, and who we are becoming.

EQUITY IN CONTEXTS

As technology continues to improve and disrupt our healthcare system, and as we pay attention to problematic assumptions in pursuit of compassionate care, we can still move in a direction that will endeavour to better our individual and collective well-being. We can move toward equity.

While *equality* means treating everyone the same, *equity* is about treating every individual according to their needs and abilities (Kuper 2016). Equity is at the core of living together as humans and should be the foundation of our healthcare system. An equitable healthcare system would deliver appropriate and relevant care to each person and community when they need it and to where that service is most accessible.

Many in the Global North are able to seek care for their health needs; they can make a phone call to their family physician and see a provider who speaks the same language. They can attend an appointment safely and without significant risk to themselves. Increasingly, technology means they don't even need to leave their homes; they can book an appointment online or connect through web conferencing to health professionals. These healthcare systems are constructed in such a way that should make access to care both possible and safe.

Yet, even in the Global North, this seemingly attainable version of healthcare services is not attainable for everyone. Not everyone has a home, a phone, or a family doctor to call. Not everyone has access to public healthcare. Not everyone speaks the same language as their healthcare provider. Not everyone can freely visit their physician without risk to themselves. Some who need to pay for their healthcare cannot.

Certainly, there are examples of technologies developed and used to address individual inequities, such as using mobile technology for communicating with health professionals or the deployment of remote presence robotic technology (Jong, Mendez, and Jong 2019). These technologies increase equity by providing access to care within people's home communities. However, in a system where a single payer covers most healthcare costs, are we perhaps replacing human interaction with technology not because it is better for the patient, but because it is cheaper for the system? Centuries of injustice within the Global North have constructed a system that remains inequitable. In the Global South, systems of oppression, injustice, a legacy of colonialism, and in South Africa, a legacy of apartheid, similarly construct a health system where compassionate care is not accessible to all.

We argue that equity must be considered in any conceptualization and enactment of compassionate care. For us, equity is about acting with sensitivity to the unique needs of other human beings, regardless of background or individual interest (Bloom 2017). Equity is about being aware of the needs of other human beings and working toward that interest as well as, or in place of, one's own. While the basis of compassion is one's individual state of concern for another's suffering, the basis of equity is the added understanding that suffering is socially situated and structured in relationships of power. Each situation is different, and even if one can act to alleviate the suffering for one individual, the same desire or action may not alleviate the suffering of another. Even in places where compassionate care can be achieved, without equity for all, compassionate care is limited to only a privileged few. In the following section, we provide a few accounts of equity-seeking movements and describe some complexities that arise while seeking equitable compassionate care. To illustrate what we mean by equity-seeking movements, we provide three examples: Indigenous health in Canada, Women's health, and HIV/AIDS.

Equity in the Context of Indigenous Health

Indigenous peoples who have lived on the land called Canada long before it was ever given that name continue to experience poorer health outcomes, shorter life expectancies, higher infant mortality rates, and higher rates of diabetes, tuberculosis, and suicide than their non-Indigenous counterparts (Philpott 2018). From the times of first contact to the residential school system and the Sixties Scoop (First Nations Studies Program 2009), to even now, when those of us who are settlers still live on Indigenous land and when many Indigenous communities in Canada lack access to clean water and other basic infrastructure, calls for equity are needed. Indigenous communities continue to work toward and call for equity, but some non-Indigenous Canadians refuse to hear them. Ongoing racism and colonial practices undermine both the health outcomes of Indigenous peoples and their rights to self-determination (Adams 1975). Even in a country such as Canada, where a prime minister advocates on a global scale for gender equality (Trudeau 2018), continued colonialism and structural racism create persistent inequities. Our tendency, perhaps, as Canadians is to believe in the myth that Canada is a country where basic needs are met, dignity to all is granted, and equity is not far off. In doing so, we are in danger of averting our gaze from past and present realities.

Indigenous leaders, Indigenous health professionals, and allies they have identified are working to solve these health inequities. After significant effort and decades-long advocacy by Indigenous health groups, the Indigenous Health Network wrote the *Joint Commitment to Action on Indigenous Health* (Writing Working Group on behalf of the Indigenous Health Network 2019). This commitment, now ratified, commits all seventeen Canadian medical schools to developing meaningful relationships with Indigenous communities, providing resources to address institutional, epistemic, and personally mediated acts of racism within institutional cultures. It also commits the schools to admitting a minimum number of First Nations, Métis, and Inuit students each year through a robust and culturally appropriate process. This landmark framework for Indigenous health education, if fully implemented, will aid in addressing systemic injustice, institutional barriers, and bias against Indigenous peoples, and will help increase access to safe, effective, equitable, culturally safe compassionate care.

Indigenous health leaders and practitioners are also effecting change in clinical environments. For example, structures for Indigenous self-determination in health are created through health transfer agreements such as the 2018 Nishnawbe Aski Nation's agreement with the federal and provincial governments, which will restore "accountability, responsibility and resource allocation" of healthcare back to the community (Nishnawbe Aski Nation 2019, 3). A set of "wise practices" to address reconciliation and achieve equity in the context of the health system has also been put forward and is gaining awareness and traction (Richardson and Murphy 2018).

Equity in the Context of Women's Health

Another health gap in Canada exists between men and women (Women's College Hospital 2018). More women than men live below the poverty line. Women who live in marginalized communities live shorter lives and have more health problems than men. Women with lower incomes have higher instances of hypertension, heart disease, arthritis, diabetes, and substance use disorders. Many women continue to face stigma in accessing healthcare because of cultural or social circumstances (Women's College Hospital 2018). Violence against women remains an area in need of urgent attention. In a multi-national study, women who reported one incident of violence against them by a partner also reported poorer health with higher levels of emotional distress, suicidal thoughts, and suicidal attempts than non-abused women (Ellsberg, Henrica, et al. 2008). Coupled with the situation that places many women at a significant disadvantage in terms of their health, there is also a gap in health research. Globally, until the 1990s, women were not usually included in healthcare studies and medical research (Women's College Hospital 2018). Although improving, data is still reported in aggregate with too little analyses of outcomes by sex, gender, or both, despite differences in physiology and experiences of illness (Avery and Clark 2016; Day, Mason, et al. 2016). A recent study across about 2,500 journals referenced in two large psychology databases demonstrates that there is even a bias against research in gender bias (Cislak, Formanowicz, and Saguy 2018).

An equitable system would bridge the gap in the difference in health outcomes between men and women. Certainly, some efforts are being made to narrow this gap. For example, health outcomes are beginning to be reported by both sex and gender. There are focused efforts to recruit women for clinical drug trials and calls for disaggregating data by sex and gender at all stages within those trials (Tannenbaum and

Day 2017). Such changes would lessen the gap in one regard, but systemic change is required to eradicate the health gap entirely. Women still face inequities in healthcare, and women who identify with multiple equity-seeking groups face these inequities even more. Intersectional (Carbado, Williams Crenshaw, et al. 2013) approaches are needed to ameliorate or eradicate the health gap. For example, one can factor in race, gender, socio-economic status, sexual orientation, and ability, to name but a few. If only defined by, for example, a white settler upper middle-class academic, compassionate care may be limited only to those who are similarly privileged. Since our perspectives are only partial, attention needs to be paid to intersectional perspectives on healthcare and health research even beyond sex and gender. Amid this complex arena of compassion, technology, and equity are examples of inequity on the global scale, stemming from historical systems of colonization that sustain injustice.

Equity in the Context of HIV/AIDS

Here we present an example of multi-level inequity in healthcare: the comparison of HIV/AIDS in Canada and South Africa. The arrival and success of antiretroviral therapy (ART) has led some to consider HIV infection as a potential chronic disease rather than a life-ending diagnosis (Deeks, Lewin, and Havlir 2013). In Canada, HIV/AIDS rates of diagnosis are declining and remain lower than average compared to many other countries (Bourgeois, Edmunds, et al. 2017; Jonah, Bourgeois, et al. 2017). In South Africa, while still high, HIV/AIDS rates of diagnosis are also declining (UNAIDS 2018).

Timely access to ART can decrease the chances of transmission (Andrews, Wood, et al. 2012), but structural barriers such as poverty, stigma, and challenges to safe disclosure of status (O'Brien, Greene, et al. 2017) prevent some people from seeking ART in a timely manner (Kendall, Shoemaker, et al. 2018). In Canada, access to ART is generally well supported. In South Africa, by comparison, while HIV testing and access to ART are also widely available, structural barriers impede the uptake of ART and contribute to high infection rates of both HIV and the associated multidrug-resistant tuberculosis as well as poor treatment adherence. These structural barriers, some emanating from socio-cultural and historical determinants (Sileo, Fielding-Miller, et al. 2018), create complex challenges for health equity initiatives in the country. There is significant social and community stigma against those with HIV/AIDS, and this prevents people from seeking testing. In the mostly collectivist community groups in South Africa, low income patients are highly dependent on family and community members for care, support, and facilitating access to treatment sites. If the affected person is the main income earner, it affects the livelihood and status of the family. Thus, a diagnosis of HIV places a burden on an entire family, not just one individual.

In order to decrease the rates of transmission of HIV/AIDS and improve the lives of those who have these diagnoses, these examples must be approached with an equity lens. Rather than assuming one solution to HIV testing will suit all, context-based, evidence-informed approaches must be sought. In one study, text messaging was used to communicate with women living with HIV in rural areas in Canada, sending them notifications once a week to ask how they were. Those who responded with "not okay" then received a follow-up phone call by a study nurse. This study showed that using text messaging improved HIV medication adherence (King, Kinvig, et al. 2017); however, a similar approach taken in a different context did not appear to have the same results (Christopoulos, Cunningham, et al. 2017). In South Africa, there is also evidence that cellphone messaging may be a useful tool for post-partum women living with HIV in order to decrease the rates of mother-to-child transmission (Mogoba, Phillips, et al. 2019). Equity is a complex issue, needing intersectional approaches to even begin to represent our partial perspectives. Very targeted initiatives, deliberately intersectional in their approach, show some ability to encourage people with newly diagnosed HIV to seek care (Dorward, Mabuto, et al. 2017).

Health policy-makers would be wise to understand the intersections equity-seeking groups face that may prevent compassionate care from being delivered or received. While offering a blanket approach and increasing access to HIV testing may help in some areas, it may still achieve nothing without facing all the underlying complex social and structural factors as well. Otherwise, stigma will just continue to manifest.

Smith (2008) notes that one way in which equity has been embraced in the search for new medicines in ethnobotany, for example, is through a code of ethics that was developed with Indigenous participation. Similar guidelines or codes of engagement could be drafted in many examples where we seek to eliminate health gaps, maybe particularly so in areas with deeply rooted stigma such as HIV prevention and care. Equity must precede compassion, particularly in situations where the most vulnerable populations face systemic health gaps. One way to bring this equity lens to your work is through reflective practice.

REFLECTIVE PRACTICE

Different people define reflective practice in different ways (Naidu and Kumagai 2016), but for the purposes of this chapter we will use the following definition: it is "a formalized 'way of doing' that includes reflection (i.e., thinking during or after doing), critical reflection (i.e., reflection to connect individual identity and social context), and reflexivity" (i.e., introspection and collaboration toward the critical analysis of social conditions and injustice) (Kumagai and Naidu 2015, 283). Reflective practice demands paying attention to another individual and realizing that we operate in relation to one another. If being compassionate means acting on one's awareness of another's suffering, then reflective practice should be an enabling feature toward equity and compassionate care itself. If being compassionate means community and collective engagement first, then reflective practice would offer insight into privilege, power, justice, and injustice. Reflective practitioners connect themselves to others in society in a meaningful and purposeful way. Reflective practitioners may be able to see how technology can be applied equitably by consulting with communities and patients and not merely applying their own individual understanding to a concern. Inequity is not overturned solely by reflection, though; there must be action taken to achieve change.

Freire (2000) and Biko (2015) are two examples of individuals who developed reflective practice as a means to tackle inequities. Through their own reflections on compassion, or their observations about the lack of compassion, they acted empathetically on their feelings and produced change in their communities. Their work alerted those around them to structural injustice and systemic inequities. The result was that they were both arrested in their respective countries of Brazil and South Africa, and Biko was murdered for his actions.

Freire's book *Pedagogy of the Oppressed* is of particular use in establishing reflective practice. In this work, he critiques what he calls the "banking model" of education, where a teacher just deposits knowledge into a passive learner. Instead he suggests that educators should use "problem-posing" education, forcing the learner to be active in their own learning process and to engage in a free and equal exchange between themselves and their teacher (Freire 2000). This transformational process leads to a shift in power: the teacher becomes a learner and the learner becomes a teacher. Through transformational education and dialogue, we develop *conscientização*, or critical consciousness. It is an equalizing and liberating form of education. Neither the learner nor the teacher is ever "fixed" or static, but instead, both are continually developing and are always unfinished.

Freire calls for reflection and action in order to transform the world. He suggests that through critical consciousness, we reflect on what we have learned and experienced and then develop actions to transform our reality. He calls this process *praxis* (Freire 2000). Unlike reflection, praxis leads to social change. Through developing perception in praxis, one sees a situation from a different perspective and then works to alter that reality for the betterment of others, thereby challenging both privilege and oppression.

In the example of healthcare, Freire's work has been used to help understand perspectives other than one's own, appreciate the context of individual learners, and recognize one's own privilege (Halman, Baker, and Ng 2017). It has been used to critique existing power structures, challenge norms, resist the status quo, and identify one's own agency. Healthcare providers need to engage in critical consciousness-raising and praxis to work toward equity, acknowledging that with privilege comes a responsibility to enact social change. To be a truly compassionate practitioner, one must be a reflective practitioner, recognizing the need for social justice and acting to improve it. Advocates for equity have pushed for structural reform to health policies, promoted people with perspectives different from their own to lead change, and handed over authority to those communities with the most to gain or lose from a decision.

When faced with new technology, reflective practitioners will begin with an understanding that technology as a practice is messy, and when ideas emerge into the real world, they do not automatically serve everyone equitably. Reflection and action will help define and then *continuously redefine* compassion and compassionate care so that those who have the power to change the system can embrace multiple and evolving perspectives. These actions can help ensure that a singular worldview is not the only one represented in one's work, policy, or practice.

Compassionate care comes only when it is distributed equitably. Otherwise, the needs of the many overwhelm the compassion for the few. As health workers and leaders, scholars and community members, we need to strive to increase compassionate care, either with or without technology, in an equitable way. Reflective practitioners will know that compassionate care will not be established with technology alone, but if deployed with a focus on equity and equitable distribution, compassionate care can be more easily realized. Solutions could include ethical guidelines for work that are developed by or co-developed with the communities they should seek to serve. Critical reflection may help identify the perspectives that need to be considered in one's work. If we move forward without the recognition of partial perspectives, without an understanding of how technologies change how we work, and without a focus on equity, both for individuals and for entire communities, compassionate care will only be fully enacted for the lucky few.

PART TWO

Cultivating Compassion

4

Healthcare Workers as Recipients of Compassion: Resilience, Burnout, and Relationship

Robert Maunder, Deanna Chaukos, and Andrea Lawson

When Dr Shelly Dev went public about her experience of burnout, she described the pressure she felt to discharge patients from hospital as quickly as possible instead of when they were ready to go home, and her subsequent anger at these patients when they would return. She recalled "feeling so distant from the reasons behind why I actually became a doctor" (CBC Radio 2018). The profound loss of professional identity that Dr Dev described is shared by many healthcare workers who lose their sensitivity to patients and find their desire to alleviate their patients' suffering to wane as a result of burnout. The introduction to this book cites a common definition of compassion as "sensitivity to the pain or suffering of another, coupled with a deep desire to alleviate that suffering" (Seppälä, Simon-Thomas, et al. 2017). Compassion is intrinsic to the work and identity of healthcare providers and is directly compromised by burnout.

Some of the conditions that lead to burnout are inherent in healthcare work, which often involves a desire to alleviate suffering that cannot be alleviated. Despite the *Oxford Dictionary*'s (2009) definition of medicine as "the science or practice of the diagnosis, treatment, and prevention of disease," most of the actual practice of medicine (and more broadly, the practice of healthcare) concerns issues that extend beyond these activities. Most healthcare dollars and hours are focused on chronic diseases that can be treated but are not usually prevented and cannot be cured (Pfuntner, Wier, and Stocks 2013). Indeed, healthcare often consists of managing the complexity that accompanies the suffering of patients who have multiple chronic illnesses that can only be partially controlled. Many of the elements of this complexity lie beyond the reach of expert medical knowledge, technical skill, or biological innovation and yet pull at healthcare professionals' desire to alleviate suffering. When one takes a compassionate approach to suffering that cannot be sufficiently alleviated, it has personal costs.

Furthermore, patients' complex chronic medical conditions often occur in the context of financial strain, social isolation, and various types of social and cultural marginalization (Marmot 2015; Schaink, Kuluski, et al. 2012). Leo Eisensten, a medical student writing in the *New England Journal of Medicine*, describes how clinicians "may feel worn down by the poverty and oppression their patients face; may feel powerless [to help] and feel demoralized when they realize that their instruction 'Do not take this medication on an empty stomach' translates into patients taking their medications only sporadically because they don't have enough to eat" (Eisenstein 2018, 519).

Processes that frustrate healthcare workers' desire for autonomy and control in the service of their patients' well-being are potent contributors to burnout. The need to contain costs drives measures that interfere with compassionate care, such as the pressure that Dr Dev felt to discharge patients prematurely. As complex presentations of chronic illnesses become more common, the cost of their treatments rises quickly. In 2011, the Harvard School of Public Health's Global Economic Forum estimated the cost of chronic non-infectious diseases in the United States alone over the following twenty years to be an absolutely unsustainable $47 trillion (Bloom, Cafiero, et al. 2011). To put that number in context, at the time of the estimate, this projected cost equalled three-quarters of the gross domestic product of the entire planet and was enough to eradicate two dollars per day poverty for the 2.5 billion people on Earth living in that condition for fifty years. Technological advances, such as electronic medical records (EMRS), have also had a substantial negative impact on healthcare workers' autonomy and control, which we discuss at length below.

Much of this book focuses on compassion directed by healthcare providers toward patients. In this chapter, we shift that focus toward healthcare professionals themselves. When those who have trained in the helping professions are unable to help sufficiently, when their compassion is thwarted, whether because of limitations inherent in healthcare work, or because of the imposition of unwieldy information systems or unsafe working conditions or societal conditions, how do healthcare providers suffer, and how can their suffering be prevented or remedied? These are our questions.

Simply put, healthcare is hard and healthcare workers have traditionally been providers, rather than recipients, of compassionate care. The purpose of this chapter is to understand the need for compassion *toward healthcare providers* and what forms a compassionate approach to healthcare work might take. Although our purpose does not extend to examining how healthcare workers' stress or burnout interferes with providing compassionate care to patients, it clearly does. Reducing the suffering of healthcare workers interrupts a vicious circle in which healthcare providers' empathy to patients' suffering may contribute to burnout, which results in failures of compassion, and more suffering.

THE NATURE OF THE PROBLEM

Burnout among healthcare professionals has become widely recognized. Indeed, even suicide among physicians is disturbingly common. Dr Pamela Wible, who experienced suicidal thoughts while feeling disillusioned about practicing medicine, describes how her reflections during a colleague's funeral led her to collect the stories of over 1,200 doctors who died by suicide (CBC Radio 2019).

Stress and resilience among professionals have also become prominent in the academic healthcare literature. Our search yielded approximately 2,000 academic contributions about interventions for burnout alone, indicating widespread concern about the problem. However, at first pass, this work does not yield coherent themes. It refers to overlapping but somewhat different constructs, such as depression, burnout, vicarious traumatization, and compassion fatigue, without any clear organizing framework. It sometimes fails to make critical distinctions, such as the distinction between depressive symptoms (which are universal) and depressive disorders (which are mental illnesses). This literature is much more often descriptive than explanatory and very rarely prescriptive.

Despite these inconsistencies, two key facts emerge. First, *the prevalence of burnout is high*. Burnout, as it is usually conceptualized (Maslach, Jackson, and Leitner 1997), consists of three components: emotional exhaustion, a sense of diminished personal connection to people and things (called depersonalization), and a diminished sense of personal accomplishment. Almost all studies of burnout measure emotional exhaustion, which includes perceptions of being overextended and drained; some studies also measure the other two components. Measured this way, the prevalence of burnout in nurses, doctors, and trainees is at least 25 per cent in most settings and sometimes substantially higher (Adriaenssens, de Gucht, and Maes 2015; Monsalve-Reyes, San Luis-Costa, et al. 2018; Dyrbye, West, et al. 2014; Trufelli, Bensi, et al. 2008; Soler, Yaman, et al. 2008). In a 2016 Mayo Clinic survey of 7,000 physicians, more than half reported burnout.

Second, *burnout has adverse consequences for patients and healthcare providers*. Burnout has been associated with many adverse effects. These include an increase in healthcare providers' sick days and other forms of lost productivity (Crowe, Bower, et al. 2018; Dewa, Loong, et al. 2014), as well as a range of mental health problems including anxiety, depression, substance use disorders, and suicidal thoughts (Ahola and Hakanen 2007; Oreskovich, Kaups, et al. 2012; Shanafelt, Dyrbye, et al. 2011). One study observed that medical students experiencing burnout performed worse on tests of medical knowledge (West, Shanafelt, and Kolars 2011), and another observed that resident physicians with burnout exhibited poorer cognitive reasoning abilities (Durning, Costanza, et al. 2013). Not surprisingly, given those correlations, burnout in healthcare providers is also associated with both self-reported and objective errors, reduced patient safety, and decreased patient satisfaction (Salyers, Bonfils, et al. 2017; Hall, Johnson, et al. 2016; Lu, Weygandt, et al. 2018; Panagioti, Geraghty, et al. 2018). A recent meta-analysis found that burnout doubles the odds of physicians being involved in incidents that put patient safety at risk (Panagioti, Geraghty, et al. 2018). Indeed, high patient-nurse ratio, an important antecedent of nursing burnout, is associated with increased patient mortality (Aiken, Clarke, et al. 2002).

To develop a more coherent understanding of workplace stress, and to consider strategies for directing compassion toward healthcare providers, we will be selective in our review of prior work. Our approach is to favour synthesis over analysis, to emphasize the themes that emerge from this body of work, and to privilege certain of those themes because they are directly relevant to compassionate care. One of these themes is that many of the sources of stress in healthcare work are interpersonal, especially conflict, isolation, violence, and gradients of power and class. By the same token, powerful sources of resilience are also interpersonal: social support, teamwork, and just distributions of power and decision-making authority. In keeping with this theme, we discuss stress and resilience with special attention to what happens for better or worse *between* people who work in healthcare. Another emerging theme, which is also a focus of this book, is the potential of technology either to exacerbate or to alleviate workplace stress.

CAUSES OF BURNOUT

Some sources of stress apply to virtually all occupations. Working in *high-demand/low-control* conditions is known to reduce well-being, especially when social support is also low (Siegrist 1996). Such environments are common in healthcare, and they have been shown to have negative effects on nurses (Lee, Lee, et al. 2014; Wendsche, Hacker, et al. 2016; van Doorn, van Ruyssevldt, et al. 2016). Similarly, *high-effort/low-reward* conditions contribute to workplace stress in many occupations, including healthcare (Padilla Fortunatti and Palmeiro-Silva 2017). Considering the components of burnout, it is easy to imagine that an environment with high demands and little control over one's work could lead to emotional exhaustion. Similarly, making great effort without receiving sufficient rewards is very likely to diminish one's sense of personal accomplishment. Shift work and overly long shifts, both common in healthcare, have also been shown to reduce well-being in many settings (Portoghese, Galletta, et al. 2014; Wisetborisut, Angkurawaranon, et al. 2014; Dall'Ora, Griffiths, et al. 2015).

Other universal sources of occupational stress are inherently social or interpersonal. The Whitehall II Study demonstrated that relatively modest *gradients of power or class* between groups of people who work in the same environment (in this case between employment grades in the British civil service) are associated with a wide range of adverse health outcomes, including mortality in the lower status groups (Marmot, Smith, et al. 1991). This is an important finding, in part because even members of the disadvantaged classes in this study had secure employment and adequate access to healthcare; the health risks relate to gradients of power and status, not to poverty or barriers to medical attention.

A related but less well-known occupational condition that *supports* well-being is *organizational justice*, which includes both a procedural component ("the extent to which decision-making processes include input from affected parties, are consistently applied, suppress bias, and are accurate, correctable and ethical") and a relational component ("polite, considerate and fair treatment of individuals") (Kivimaki, Elovainio, et al. 2003, 27). For hospital employees, lower levels of organizational justice are associated with poor self-rated health, psychiatric symptoms, and sick days (Elovainio, Kivimaki, and Vahtera 2002). Remarkably, in primary care health centres, healthcare providers' perceptions of greater organizational justice were also associated with better glycemic control in their patients with type II diabetes (Virtanen, Oksanen, et al. 2012).

Deficits in *social support* are clearly important in the development of burnout because support may both improve well-being directly and buffer the impact stressors (Cohen and Syme 1985). However, it matters *who* is providing the support. Support from family, colleagues, and supervisors may be more effective than support from other sources (W. Stroebe, M. Stroebe, and Abakoumkin 1996). Different kinds of support (e.g., emotional versus practical) may affect different aspects of burnout (Halbesleben 2006).

Other sources of stress are unique to healthcare. *Exposure to violence* from patients is a remarkably common experience, especially for nurses. More than a third of nurses report exposure to workplace physical violence, often with injury (Spector, Zhou, and Che 2014). The majority of nurses report being bullied or verbally abused at work, especially by physicians and patients (Spector, Zhou, and Che 2014; Felblinger 2011). These behaviours can have a direct impact on patient safety and the quality of care. For example, nurses report that bullying interferes with clarity in dispensing medication (Institute for Safe Medication Practices 2004).

Healthcare also exposes workers to other types of trauma and critical incidents. Some of these, including extraordinary outbreaks of infectious diseases such as SARS, temporarily affect a wide range of healthcare workers (Shanafelt, Sloan, and Habermann 2003; Maunder, Lancee, et al. 2006). Others are inherent to the work of specific groups, such as paramedics (Crowe, Bower, et al. 2018). Certain specialties are associated with a greater risk of burnout, including emergency medicine, general internal medicine, neurology, family medicine, and emergency nursing (Hooper, Craig, et al. 2010). Some identify repeated exposure to patients'·trauma, which is often referred to as vicarious traumatization, as a contributor to burnout, although the evidence is mixed (Makadia, Sabin-Farrell, and Turpin 2017; Sinclair and Hamill 2007).

For resident physicians (trainees), five primary contributors to burnout have been identified: (1) inadequate work support, (2) work inefficiency (with emerging themes around chaos as a potent contributor), (3) loss of workplace autonomy, (4) challenges to work-life balance, and (5) loss of meaning in one's work (Shanafelt, Sloan, and Habermann 2003; Krasner, Epstein, et al. 2009). The experience of being both under-supported *and* under-equipped might make resident physicians uniquely prone to burnout (Benson, Chaukos, et al. 2018). The loss of meaning in work is another area in which vicious feedback cycles may occur, as lost meaning may be both a cause and consequence of burnout.

One also has to look beyond the characteristics of the workplace to consider how stress and resilience are related to the individual characteristics of healthcare professionals and their social context. Although individual characteristics are an important part of a comprehensive understanding of burnout, we should be careful not to blame the victim (Shanafelt 2018). Younger age (and therefore inexperience), female gender, less education, and lower socio-economic status may increase vulnerability to the adverse consequences of work stress (Amoafo, Hanbali, et al. 2015; Ayalon 2008; Canadas-De la Fuente, Vargas, et al. 2015; Soares, Grossi, and Sundin 2007).

Prior exposure to trauma is a risk factor for most stress response syndromes (Brewin, Andrews, and Valentine 2000), and so probably also for burnout, although information about prior personal traumas is often not surveyed in studies of healthcare professionals' burnout. Consistent with this hypothesis, we found that a history of childhood abuse or neglect was associated with higher levels of burnout in paramedics (Maunder, Halpern, et al. 2012). Trauma is of particular importance because it is so common. The majority of adults have been exposed to adversity with potential health consequences as children (Gilbert, Breiding, et al. 2015). Looking beyond developmental trauma, 25 per cent of female nurses report intimate partner violence and about 23 per cent report emotional abuse by an intimate partner (Bracken, Messing, et al. 2010). There is a compelling argument that "wounded healers" may seek out careers in healing professions, where past resilience to adverse experiences may contribute to compassionate and patient-centred care (Gallop, McKeever, et al. 1995).

The evidence about differential rates of past adversity in healthcare workers and in the general population is, however, inconsistent. In our research, for example, the rate of childhood trauma among hospital workers was high (33 per cent), but not necessarily higher than that found in the general population (Maunder, Peladeau, et al. 2010), whereas the rate among paramedics was significantly elevated (male 35 per cent, female 44 per cent) (Maunder, Halpern, et al. 2012). Current and past trauma may increase vulnerability to stressors, whether or not healthcare workers are at higher risk than other members of their communities.

THE IMPACT OF THE ELECTRONIC MEDICAL RECORD AND INFORMATION SYSTEMS

In recent years, two forces have combined to change the workday tasks of healthcare professionals. One is the introduction of EMRs. The second is the increasing emphasis on measurement in the service of quality improvement and cost containment (Porter and Teisberg 2006). Many of the administrative tasks associated with EMRs and implementation of evidence-based quality measures have been downloaded to clinicians, with insufficient regard for flow, efficiency, and downstream costs (Shanafelt, Dyrbye, et al. 2016). The amount of work that this has generated is staggering: up to two hours of administrative work for each hour of direct patient care, much of it completed from home on weeknights and weekends (Arndt, Beasley, et al. 2017). In a thoughtful essay on the impact of EMRs on physicians, Gawande (2018a, 65) describes this burden of time, but also how EMRs make gathering information about patients less efficient as healthcare professionals navigate "this massive monster of incomprehensibility" that results from lack of attention to quality improvement strategies to streamline processes within the EMR software (Shanafelt, Dyrbye, and West 2017; Thomas, Ripp, and West 2018). These processes of digital data collection and communication are striking examples of high-demand/low-control and high-effort/low-reward activities introduced into professions that have historically enjoyed both high control and high reward.

More insidiously, the computer interface required for EMRs may lead to interpersonal disconnection. Even when it increases efficiency, the presence of the EMR screen interferes with patient-physician communication (Shachak, Hadas-Dayagi, et al. 2009). Gawande observes disconnection between colleagues as well as patients: "The software changed how people work together. They'd become more disconnected; less likely to see and help one another, and often less able to" (Gawande 2018a, 66).

Thus, technology that has been introduced to improve the quality and value of healthcare may bring with it several factors that increase the risk of burnout: high demand/low control, high effort/low reward, interpersonal disconnection, and challenges to work-life balance. For healthcare professionals doing work that is inherently challenging, EMRS add burden and reduce opportunities to provide compassionate care to patients. Institutional requirements to use EMRS may exemplify the pressures to work in ways that erode professional identity, which Dr Dev found were driving her feelings of burnout.

WHAT WE CAN LEARN FROM MAGNET HOSPITALS

In 1983, McLure, Poulin, and Sovie (1983) observed that nurses considered certain hospitals good places to work, and so these institutions had lower staff turnover. They designated these institutions Magnet hospitals. Subsequent research demonstrates that Magnet hospitals have better patient outcomes, including lower patient mortality (Aiken, Smith, and Lake 1994). The characteristics that distinguish Magnet hospitals reveal strategies for building more compassionate work environments.

These are the characteristics of Magnet hospitals: a formal organizational structure that is relatively flat (fewer supervisors), a nurse among the hospital's top executives, autonomy for nurses to make clinical decisions within their area of competence and to control their practice, decentralized decision-making, adequate staffing, and a culture that recognizes the importance of nursing (through salaries rather than hourly wages, support for continuing education, and supportive supervisors) (Aiken, Smith, and Lake 1994). Taken as a whole, these characteristics are associated with the empowerment of nurses within the workplace (Laschinger, Almost, and Tuer-Hodes 2003). Not surprisingly, nurses in Magnet hospitals have greater job satisfaction and less burnout (Bracken, Messing, et al. 2010).

Magnet hospitals appear to establish a better balance of demand and control, reduce gradients of power between professional disciplines, pursue organizational justice, and provide social support. Thus, these institutions embody many of the characteristics that evidence supports as buffering occupational stress.

Currently, Magnet status, accompanied by the symbol of a registered trademark in particular contexts, is an official designation awarded by the American Nurses Credentialing Center, an affiliate of the

American Nurses Association. Appraisal of an institution to gain
Magnet recognition is extensive and expensive. It has been criticized
as a designation that serves the marketing of designated hospitals
more than it serves their staff or patients. Nevertheless, the characteristics of Magnet hospitals that led to their identification in the first
place remain instructive. They serve as an effective argument that
hospitals, as institutions, can support the well-being of their staff
through their choices about policies and organizational structure.

WHAT WE CAN LEARN FROM SARS

We studied how the extraordinary stress of working through a several-
month outbreak of SARS affected hospital workers in Toronto, Canada.
At the time of its emergence in Toronto in February 2003, the coro-
navirus that caused SARS was unknown. The outbreak was spreading
around the world at an unprecedented rate. An alarming number of
healthcare workers were themselves becoming infected and dying.
In the first wave of the outbreak, infection control procedures were
inadequate and mortality from infection appeared to be high. Although
effective infection control procedures subsequently reduced the rate
of transmission substantially, the experience of working in a hospital
with affected patients (often colleagues who had become infected)
was exceptionally stressful (Maunder, Lancee, et al. 2005).

We found that interpersonal factors were strongly associated both
with markedly high rates of acute stress and with severe long-term
stress responses. One of the more potent of the acute contributors
to stress was interpersonal isolation (Maunder, Lancee, et al. 2005).
Quarantine practices were the most obvious but not the only form
of interpersonal distancing. Interacting with patients required donning
protective equipment, including gowns, masks, gloves, and face shields.
One patient said during rounds that she had taken to memorizing the
shoes that her nurses and doctors wore because there was no other
way to identify who was entering her room when the always-closed
door swung open.

Healthcare workers also had less contact with each other. To reduce
the risk of contagion, they were instructed to minimize contact with
colleagues by, for example, maintaining extra space between individuals and cancelling non-essential group meetings. Outside the
workplace, many healthcare workers chose to maintain distance from
loved ones, or they were avoided by members of their families and

communities. The latter form of social disconnection became especially apparent as the first wave of the outbreak continued through Easter and Passover (Maunder, Hunter, et al. 2003; Maunder, Lancee, et al. 2005). Since social support is known to be one of the most effective buffers of stress, the numerous ways in which healthcare can interfere with support circumstances such as these can be a powerful impediment to resilience.

Some healthcare professionals were more affected by these conditions than others. To understand why, we turned to interpersonal psychology. We particularly turned to attachment theory, which is a useful framework for understanding these dynamics because it is a robustly evidence-supported theory of close interpersonal relationships; it is directly relevant to both the value of interpersonal support and its limitations; and it describes normal psychology rather than pathology. Links between variations in attachment dynamics and variations in vulnerability to stress are well established (Maunder and Hunter 2001; Maunder and Hunter 2015).

Feeling secure in our relationships with those closest to us is the interpersonal base from which compassion is most effective. Different patterns of adult attachment represent normal variations in how we relate to those closest to us in order to feel as secure as possible as often as possible. Insecure patterns of attachment can be described in terms of attachment anxiety (a need for closer relationships and dependency) and attachment avoidance (a preference for more distant relationships and independence). In hospital workers, we found that both dimensions of attachment insecurity were correlated with poor sleep quality and physical symptoms, while attachment anxiety was also related to sick days and depressive symptoms (Maunder, Hunter, and Lancee 2011). In paramedics, we found that the combination of both types of insecurity was correlated with slow recovery from critical incidents, depressive symptoms, and burnout (Halpern, Maunder, et al. 2012).

Compassionate support for healthcare workers needs to be aligned with individual preferences for support and attentive to the quality of interpersonal networks in the workplace. The attachment perspective brings a helpful focus to these aspects of the interpersonal environment, rather than the emphasis on individual vulnerability or resilience, which permeates much of the literature on burnout. For example, attachment theory teaches us that all individuals thrive best (take chances, explore, create, and learn) in such circumstances that they are reasonably assured of a "secure base" to work from. The workplace environment that would provide a secure base is likely quite closely aligned with principles of organizational justice (reliable, transparent, and fair processes for managing interpersonal dynamics), emotional support (relationships with trusted and supportive colleagues and mentors), and some characteristics of Magnet hospitals (the security of salaried work rather than hourly wages). Furthermore, attachment theory emphasizes the value for resilience of very close, reciprocal, confidante relationships outside the workplace, which often are found in committed romantic relationships. This helps explain why hospital workers who were single (not living with a partner) were at higher risk of the long-term effects of stress while working during the SARS outbreak.

With respect to individual differences, attachment theory suggests wide variance in the patterns of seeking and receiving help that make a person feel most secure. This perspective has allowed us to encourage healthcare workers to individualize their coping strategies by knowing themselves and what works best for them. For example, we encourage colleagues to talk to others and seek support if it helps, without feeling obligated to do so if open discussion of vulnerable emotions feels aversive.

IMPROVING THE WELL-BEING
OF HEALTHCARE WORKERS

Our review has emphasized how burnout is increased by interpersonal disconnection, interpersonal harm, high-demand/low-control environments, and high-effort/low-reward environments. We have pointed out the potential for poorly designed EMRs to contribute to these harms, and the potential for workplaces with the characteristics of Magnet hospitals to ameliorate them. Unfortunately, randomized controlled trials (RCTs) of interventions to reduce burnout have, for the most part, not tested interventions designed to improve these factors. Indeed, it is remarkable what little research has focused on how to change the workplace to preserve the health of healthcare professionals.

A systematic review of RCTs to prevent and reduce burnout in physicians (West, Dyrbye, et al. 2016) found only three RCTs that focused on changes to the structure of the work environment. These three tested the impact of shortening the length of attending physicians' rotations on a service (Lucas, Trick, et al. 2012); shortening the length of residents' shifts (Parshuram, Amaral, et al. 2015); and a mix of interventions to workflow, communication, and other aspects of work conditions (Linzer, Poplau, et al. 2015). The interventions are quite different in these three studies and results are inconsistent. Another analysis, including a wider range of studies, found that strategies targeting organizational change were more effective at preventing burnout than those targeting individuals (Panagioti, Panagopoulou, et al. 2017). The consistent focus of workplace interventions that contributed to this positive effect was scheduling of physician shifts.

Looking beyond physicians, a Cochrane review of interventions to prevent psychological stress in healthcare workers found fifty-eight RCTs, of which twenty addressed organizational interventions (Marine, Ruotsalainen, et al. 2006). Organizational interventions to change schedules (increases in days off or shorter blocks of work days) reduced stress, while other interventions (organizing support, changing care, increasing communication skills) had no effect. Thus, RCTs, which provide our most robust source of evidence of the efficacy of interventions, support the "low-hanging fruit" that reducing harmful scheduling practices reduces stress. It is time to develop and test organizational interventions that increase connection, control, and reward.

Several interventions that focus on individual resilience, rather than organizational change, have also been studied. One rationale for individual interventions is that they might protect against the known effects of the practice environment on burnout. The 2006 Cochrane review cited above, which examined interventions to prevent psychological stress in healthcare workers, found very limited evidence of benefit of cognitive behavioural therapy, mindfulness meditation, and relaxation, based on low quality data (Marine, Ruotsalainen, et al. 2006). More recent meta-analyses have examined RCTs and cohort studies of individual-level interventions to prevent or reduce burnout for physicians, including stress management, communication skills training, and mindfulness-based interventions. As a group these were less effective than organization-level interventions (Panagioti, Panagopoulou, et al. 2017) but contributed to an overall modest benefit (West, Dyrbye, et al. 2016).

Preventive strategies might be more effective if implemented earlier in a healthcare professional's career. One RCT found that first-year medical residents who participated in web-based cognitive behaviour therapy for the reduction of suicidal thoughts were 60 per cent less likely to report suicidal thoughts during their internship year (Guille, Zhou, et al. 2015). Individual preventive interventions can also be combined with organizational changes, and there is some evidence that the combination has more sustained benefits (Awa, Plaumann, and Walter 2010; Westermann, Kozak, et al. 2014).

A WIDER SCAN FOR APPROACHES TO BOLSTERING HEALTHCARE WORKERS' WELL-BEING

It is helpful to look beyond RCTs for further ideas. Looking to the experience of staff in Magnet hospitals, for example, suggests how organizations can shift toward a healthier culture and interpersonal environment by engaging members of key employee groups in the leadership team and fostering local and individual autonomy. Exploring business literature, we found an emphasis on the value of "organizational resilience" (Maunder, Leszcz, et al. 2008), which is similar to the ecological concept of resilient systems. Within resilient systems, disturbance is not only tolerated but creates possibilities for innovation and development (Folke 2006). Organizational resilience is thought to foster the individual resilience of employees and is good for business. One characteristic of organizations regarded as more resilient is having adequate reserves, which refers to material or financial reserves and also structural reserves in the form of backup plans and succession plans (Freeman, Hirschorn, and Maltz 2004; Hamel and Välikangas 2003).

Beyond material and structural reserves, we argue for the value of "relational reserves," which refers to organizations that have untapped capacity for providing interpersonal support. Social support can be a powerfully beneficial force, but experience teaches that support from colleagues or co-workers at the time of a crisis is much more effective when it occurs in the context of already existing relationships (Maunder, Hunter, et al. 2003; Maunder, Lancee, et al. 2005). During the SARS outbreak, for example, very few staff chose to attend formal support groups when they were made available, but many spoke to a psychiatrist friend for an informal "hallway consultation" to discuss insomnia or to commiserate about stress. Processes and activities that foster strong collegial relationships and social networks, creating links across disciplines and working groups, provide reserves for future interpersonal support. The benefits of that support emerge in unanticipated ways as stressors evolve. This idea of relational reserves goes well beyond traditional professional supports offered by large organizations (via, for example, Employee Assistance Programs).

The role of effective leadership in organizational resilience is complex and important. A style of organizational leadership that is perceived to be controlling has been associated with poor professional quality of life (Hiles Howard, Parris, et al. 2015). In contrast, adaptive governance is a key aspect of resilient systems, and includes leadership by persons who foster trust and provide vision and meaning (Folke, Hahn, et al. 2005; Freeman, Hirschorn, and Maltz 2004). In healthcare organizations, meaning can sometimes be found in a shared dedication to caring for the sick (Maunder, Lancee, et al. 2008), which aligns with the empirically supported value of invoking a sense of moral purpose to cope with events that do not yield to problem-solving or emotion-focused strategies to tolerate irresolvable distress (Folkman and Greer 2000). Leadership coaching that fosters perspective-taking capacity, self-insight, tolerance of ambiguity, and solution-focused thinking has been found to reduce stress and anxiety among the leaders who received the coaching (leaving unanswered for now the impact of this coaching on those within the leaders' organizations who might benefit from their learning) (Grant, Studholme, et al. 2017). These approaches are consistent with the model of compassionate leadership advanced by Tassone and colleagues in chapter 6 of this book.

There is an economic case for building compassionate organizations. Burnout drains organizational reserves by increasing turnover, decreasing productivity, compromising institutional vision, and diminishing quality and safety. Supports for workers, including leadership and professional development, promise to prevent significant waste (Shanafelt, Goh, and Sinsky 2017). Staff well-being might be considered both a quality marker and a wise organizational investment (Thomas, Ripp, and West 2018).

HARNESSING TECHNOLOGY TO BUILD RESILIENCE IN HEALTHCARE WORKERS: A CASE STUDY

Having had the unfortunate opportunity to extensively study the long-term effects of SARS on hospital workers in 2003 and 2004, we were well positioned to participate in efforts to prepare hospital staff for an influenza pandemic when one seemed imminent a few years later. The existing evidence did not give us clear guidance about what we should do, but there were some relatively clear parameters.

Tolerating extraordinary workplace stresses often means learning to live with uncertainty and suffering that cannot be changed. In this sense, challenges to resilience are greatest in situations where problem-solving is not a viable option. Healthcare workers had told us about this during SARS; intensive care nurses, for example, had told us that they had chosen their work because they are highly effective in situations that require rapid reactions and urgent problem-solving. They found it very difficult to tolerate being in a stressful situation in which such reactivity was ineffective because uncertainty was high and solutions were unavailable. They learned, they told us, that it was more adaptive to be reflective upon their situation rather than reactive to it. "Don't just do something, sit there" was a difficult lesson for healthcare workers who considered themselves experts at near-instant responses to life-and-death problems.

We had two core goals in preparing healthcare workers for the stress of a pandemic. The first was to increase their sense of comfort and skill in reflection, as opposed to immediate reaction. The second was to improve interpersonal functioning (or, framing this negatively, to reduce interpersonal problems), and thus increase their capacity for interpersonal connection. Continuing professional education research consistently shows that didactic presentations of knowledge don't change attitudes or behaviour. Instead, we needed a curriculum that involved experiential learning, practice, and, ideally, coaching. Knowing the importance of individual differences in coping, in accessing interpersonal support, and in appraisal of workplace stresses, we also wanted to develop a curriculum that was adaptable to individual needs.

Because we were preparing for a pandemic that had the potential to affect hundreds of thousands of healthcare workers, whatever we developed also had to be scalable and inexpensive to distribute. This was one pragmatic reason we focused on factors that could change at the level of individuals rather than on organizational factors; we could imagine an experiential course that could be available to thousands of health professionals in the available time, but we could not imagine changing the culture of thousands of workplaces.

The result of that work was an online, interactive training resource called the Stress Vaccine. The course was set up in a series of modules that each contained a variety of multiple short tasks and exercises. Some exercises were didactic, for example, learners were to describe common effective tactics for coping. Some exercises evaluated individual differences, for example learners were asked to complete a survey that measured coping style, or common interpersonal problems, or attachment patterns. In these cases, the program retained the information in order to select subsequent exercises to match each learner's preferences or needs. One exercise directly surveyed the types of workplace situations that the learner found most challenging. Again, the information was saved to personalize subsequent modules. Learners could practice relaxation exercises based on boxed breathing or progressive muscle relaxation, guided by audiotaped instruction.

Whatever other exercises were included, every module included one reflective, interactive video exercise. For these exercises, learners watched a brief (about one minute) professionally produced video vignette that depicted hospital scenes scripted to induce stress. For example, a patient's relative makes an angry demand that is probably well justified, but impossible to meet; a hospital worker at home is caught between the expectations of her partner and an unexpected demand from her employer; two colleagues have a dispute when one doesn't follow rules designed to control infectious risk. In every case, the video ends abruptly before resolution is possible.

The learner then completed an interactive exercise that required reflection on coping, emotions, and interpersonal dynamics. This exercise included questions such as, "How would this situation make you feel?," "What would you do next?," "Would that change how you felt?," "How might someone else react in the same situation?" Learners worked through an interactive sequence in which the next question depended on their answers to the previous one, resulting in a short, personalized find-your-own-adventure-type sequence of questions and responses. Reflective exercises were also personalized by the selection of videos from a library to match situations that learners had rated as especially challenging.

We compared different "doses" of the intervention by randomizing learners to courses composed of different numbers of modules: short (7 modules, 111 minutes), medium (12 modules, 128 minutes), or long (17 modules, 223 minutes). We found that the different doses of intervention were associated with a gradient of benefits – improved confidence in support and training, improved self-efficacy, and reduced interpersonal problems – with the optimal ratio of burden to benefit in the medium-length course (Maunder, Lancee, et al. 2010). Each of these outcomes was known from the post-SARS work to be a proximal determinant of better long-term stress outcomes. The dose-finding study provided evidence that virtual interactive training could improve outcomes that buffer the impact of healthcare workplace stressors. Fortunately for our colleagues, the expected pandemic turned out to be milder than anticipated, so there was no opportunity to put the Stress Vaccine to the ultimate test, to see if it actually reduced the adverse consequences of the workplace stresses of an infectious outbreak.

The Stress Vaccine was designed for a very specific context and purpose, not as a generally applicable intervention to bolster the resilience of healthcare workers. Nonetheless, it serves as a proof of concept, indicating that personalized, interactive, experiential learning to bolster resilience to stress can be provided in a format that is fully automated and virtual, and can thus be scaled up without high costs after the initial investment in the development of the resource. It is an approach that has promise for the future, both within hospitals and in other environments.

It is interesting that the Stress Vaccine appears to have greater potential to buffer stress than other individual-level interventions have shown thus far. We think this may be because of the skills it targets – building reflective skills to tolerate what cannot be immediately resolved and improving interpersonal function – and because it is a highly personalized, experiential learning resource. The Stress Vaccine also differs from other interventions in that learners could proceed through the course at their own pace. An important caveat, of course, is that a dose-finding study is not an RCT, and so the Stress Vaccine has not yet received the degree of scrutiny that has revealed the weaknesses of other individual interventions to prevent burnout.

SUMMARY

Healthcare workers usually choose their profession, in part, because they are drawn to the opportunity to show compassion to those who suffer. The rising prevalence of burnout and other consequences of workplace stress emphasize the need for compassionate approaches *toward* healthcare workers as well. Our selective and synthetic review of a very broad literature on the subject emphasizes the importance of organizational and interpersonal processes both in the causes of burnout and in the changes that are most likely to prevent it.

Compassion toward healthcare workers, in this sense, involves just processes, security, the ability to influence workplace conditions, reward that is commensurate with effort, relationships that provide support and sustenance, and effective leadership. The inevitable increase in technology in healthcare settings can certainly contribute to stress and burnout. There is also some hope that in the future technology can be harnessed to support more compassionate ends.

5

Compassion and
Health Professional Education

Claire Mallette, Donald Rose, and Michelle Spadoni

As authors, we are mid- to late-career associate professors teaching future health practitioners in the academic setting. We have been invited to write this chapter on emerging technologies in healthcare and their educational implications. Herein, we will explore the turbulence that advancing technology will generate across educational domains and within practice settings. As educators, we must not only enable learners to *use* emerging technologies – often while acquiring those skills ourselves – but also equip them to assess the various effects of those technologies in practice to ensure compassion is sustained. This challenge requires new knowledge and technical skills, as well as new identities and adaptable forms of expertise for our future health professionals to become curious, compassionate practitioners.

Our students have come of age in a world of ubiquitous technologies. Yet, we are of the Jetsons' generation. Seeds of AI were planted in our imaginations through a quirky technological cartoon created by Hanna-Barbera in the 1960s. The television show introduced our generation to moving sidewalks, laptops, rockets, and watches that monitored essential life forces. The Jetson family seamlessly interfaced with technology by doing everyday activities, such as chatting with their digital doctor, and interacting with Rosie the home android to add milk to the grocery order, which was then delivered by a flying drone to their doorstep. These items were strange futuristic ideas to us at the time; now, we can describe many of them with realistic names.

The futuristic world of the Jetsons was amplified in our memories in the summer of 1967, when Canada hosted Expo 67 in Montreal. The rail trams zooming by overhead, circling around the glass-globed America Pavilion, convinced an entire generation that technologies for the home, workspace, and health system would be the next intellectual revolution. The exhibition theme, "Man and His World," derived from *Terre des Hommes* by poet and aviator Antoine de Saint-Exupéry, was transformative for our generation through quotes such as, "It is the compelling zest of high adventure and of victory, and in creative action, that man finds his supreme joys" (de Saint-Exupéry 1950, 86).

Our generation was witness to the first organ transplants and the first man to walk on the moon. We used the first hand-held calculators and were introduced to computer hard drives that filled entire storage rooms. We remember when a cellphone was the size of a brick and weighed that much. While we dreamed of the possibilities that came in the National Aeronautics and Space Administration (NASA) era, the following generations developed the science that made possible Facebook, Instagram, Google, tablets, robotics, and the Human Genome Project.

Every new development brings the unknown and unforeseeable. Emergent technologies continue to deliver inconceivable opportunities, such as decision-making algorithms, surgical robots, and beyond. However, we must also be mindful of intended and unintended consequences that emerging technologies will have in the future, such as privacy breaches that seem beyond our view and the risk of losing the human connection in healthcare.

This is the terrain that we navigate as health profession educators. Today's student may be outpacing their teachers in relation to their technological literacy and fluency. The presence of technologies in their personal lives puts the world in their grasp with the stroke of a key or a swipe across a screen. Students in our classrooms are often more comfortable texting one another than speaking to the person beside them to discuss a question the teacher has posed. As educators we must examine what aspects of long-standing professional expertise are essential to teach and defend. Which will need to be reshaped for the better, and how will we embrace technology with creative pedagogies to teach it? As the tools of the profession change, we also need to be concerned about monitoring the effects on human relationships and fostering compassion in healthcare.

While our technologies are new, our concerns are not. Baker (2018) puts our increasing unease as teachers into perspective in his article titled "The Digital-Era Brain" for *Time* magazine's special edition on the science of memory. He recounts: "A Revolutionary New Technology was promising unprecedented access to information but was also sounding alarms: 'This invention will produce forgetfulness in the minds of those who learn to use it, because they will not practice their memory,' warned a leading mind of the era. It was 370 B.C., and the speaker was Socrates. The object of his scorn? The dreaded written word" (Baker 2018, 63).

Philosopher John Caputo (2018) provides a response that may help us address the uncertainty of educating students for a future we cannot predict in a changing healthcare environment. Caputo reminds us that it is human nature to want to flee the unknown, to swim to the safe shores of the status quo (i.e., the known). Yet, only by navigating the unknown together can we understand how uncertainty, change, and complexity are interwoven in technological systems. In healthcare, Caputo's ideas push us to explore how health professionals, educators, students, people in need of care, and families can understand and navigate uncertainty together. Caputo (1988) argues that it is only through intention, attention, and working within community that we can better see what lies ahead. How might we as educators shore up one another and draw upon one another's unique wisdom to navigate the unknown? Rather than fleeing to the safe shores of the status quo, how do we recognize these changing times as a space of possibilities while embracing in meaningful ways the turbulence of change?

Caputo's reflection is a jumping-off point for the discussion that follows. We will be exploring our concerns about preparing students for the future that we can foresee while also preparing them for the unforeseeable. Moving forward with the advancement of technology, we must face our fear, as it is in the space of possibilities and the unknown where the tensions of change, relationships, and new practices emerge. In this chapter, we will use the metaphor of crossing a turbulent river, rather than swimming to the familiar shore of the status quo, to explore how our educational practices must be responsive to technological change while ensuring compassionate care is not lost. We imagine *turbulence* as sites of uncertainty and change that technologies continually generate across educational domains: in our classrooms, practice settings, and relationships. By learning to navigate this turbulence through entering new spaces of possibility, we can strive to ensure that our future healthcare providers emerge as curious and compassionate practitioners. To achieve this, educators will need to jump into the turbulent waters, holding on to their knowledge and experience to assist in navigating the way forward, while learning to swim in new ways alongside their students, colleagues, and the people in need of care.

STANDING ON THE FAMILIAR SHORE

The riverbank of the status quo is crowded with educators, students, practitioners, and people needing care. They gaze into the turbulent waters created by technology's influence on healthcare and education, contemplating when and whether they should jump in. Some choose not to jump, believing they will be safer staying on the shore. Others have decided to jump in with a life preserver, while several are diving in head first to see where this adventure will take them. Those who enter bring different knowledge and needs that will assist or challenge them as they navigate the turbulent spaces.

Several groups remain on the shore. They include educators who believe that AI and technology will not change the role of health professionals. They hold steadfast that the knowledge and ability to care for people are irreplaceable; machines and technology will never be able to perform the roles of a nurse, physiotherapist, physician, or other health professional. They also believe that the role of an educator is the "sage on the stage" who will impart their wisdom to the students.

> ### Claire's Reflection
> Those who defend traditional approaches to education remind me of the adolescent books Helen Wells wrote in the 1940s and 50s. The book series follows a young woman, Cherry Ames, from nursing school into an exciting nursing career. As an educator, I reread the first book, *Cherry Ames Student Nurse* (1943). I was struck that Cherry's education is not very different from our current ways of teaching health professionals. On her first day, Cherry and her classmates are told that as a professional, their first duty is always to the patient. To be a nurse, they need "good health, intelligence, unselfishness, humor, sympathy … efficiency and plenty of energy for hard work" (Wells, 32). Cherry's classes

consist of anatomy and physiology, therapeutics in the effects of different medicines, patient psychology, dietetics, handwashing, spread of infection, ethics, pharmacology, obstetrics, pediatrics, and skills on a "demonstration doll" that was rubber with a "humorously resigned look on its face from suffering" (49). After hearing about all that is needed to be learned to become a nurse, Cherry exclaims, "I'm going to give up sleeping and just memorize!" (52). Her clinical experiences occurred throughout the hospital, including a coveted posting in the emergency department that was considered "the most exciting place in the hospital" (125). While our knowledge and evidence have certainly expanded in the past eighty years, if we are honest, are our educational practices or students' expectations much different than what is described in the 1940s?

As educators, we can no longer afford to teach in the same manner as we have in the past. What must we let go of or teach differently in our curricula? To answer this question, we must critically examine the knowledge, skills, and pedagogy that are now necessary for our students to become curious, compassionate practitioners for the future. Hartrick, Doane and Varcoe (2015) describe that in order for our students to be curious, they need to be encouraged to be interested, inquisitive, and open to the uncertainty of knowing and not knowing. How do we facilitate our students becoming curious and compassionate within this changing healthcare environment?

If we return to the riverbank, the people who need care are another group who stand looking at the space of possibilities. As educators and practitioners, we cannot assume that everyone is digitally literate and has access to technology. While most have access to technology, health information, and data, others will not. This can lead to both equity and ethical issues related to personalized medicine and machine-aided clinical decision-making as we move forward with the advancement of technology influencing healthcare delivery. In chapter 3, Paton and colleagues discuss these issues in much more depth and emphasize that humans must remain vigilant in ensuring the ethical and compassionate use of technology within healthcare.

The last group of people left behind on the riverbank are health practitioners who believe that they alone have the wisdom and ability needed to care for patients. When a person needs healthcare, these

clinicians decide what is best, with input from colleagues where necessary, but with little or no input from the person receiving the care.

THE JOURNEY BEGINS

Those who jump from the riverbank prepare to face the tensions of
the unknown. In the beginning, the students, educators, and practitioners remain close together. They're propelled by the desire to make
a difference and by the driving principles of empathy and compassion.
Yet, each person has their own ability to provide care and their own
understanding of empathy, shaped by their cultural backgrounds,
social environments, and past interactions with others. They bring
different perspectives and interpretations of appropriate humanistic
and compassionate behaviours (Kuper, Reeves, et al. 2007). How can
educators ensure that compassion, in all its diversity, continues to
propel them in the same direction?

The people in need of care also stay close to this group. No matter
how technology changes healthcare, they continue to want the human-
ness of empathy and compassion from their healthcare providers. Too
often, compassionate care is dismissed as small acts and kindness that
are not important or necessary. Yet, people who are cared for by health
professionals say that those uniquely human acts, such as being listened to and cared for, matter as much as the quality of the healthcare
received (Hofmeyer, Toffoli, et al. 2018). How can educators cultivate
the compassion that is so important to students, practitioners, and
people in their care? We consider this question as it relates to the
changes and uncertainties emerging within academic settings, practice
settings, relationships, and interactions with technologies themselves.

TURBULENCE IN THE ACADEMIC SETTING

Turbulence can result in the academic setting, as many faculty (ourselves included) are from a generation whose cultural interactions
and influences were very different from those of the students we teach.
We communicated by writing (or typing) on paper, speaking on the
telephone, or interacting face to face. Through these media we learned
to interpret a person's verbal and non-verbal communication and
need for compassion. This is in marked contrast from our students
who are most comfortable communicating across screens and showing emotions through emojis! How do we as educators reconcile these

modes of communication with one another and understand how compassion can be provided in ways we are unfamiliar with?

Many of us recognize that we must change our teaching practices to better meet the learning needs of our students who have learned to communicate and interpret social cues through different media. This is why we chose to jump into the river of uncertainty, holding on to a life preserver, uncomfortable with the tension of how to best teach learners of today who are so very different from us.

> ### Don's Reflection
> Recently, when I was walking to work, I looked into a Toronto streetcar going by. Inside the car, all the people sat hunched over their phones or stood bracing themselves with one hand in order to interact with their screens, unaware of their surroundings. What surprised me was that I did not observe a single conversation actually occurring face to face. Everyone was subsumed in their technology rather than engaged directly with the people around them. Yet, we presently teach our students that compassionate interactions with the people we care for should occur face to face. We must ask ourselves how this should change within the technological world, when the person who requires care may not even be in the same city.

Compassionate interaction involves a human connection with another person established through attentive listening, awareness of suffering, empathy, therapeutic communication, body language, small acts, kindness, and dignity (Durkin, Gurbutt, and Carson 2018; Richardson, Percy, and Hughes 2015). Being compassionate is a complex skill that needs to be emphasized with equal importance to learning technological and clinical skills. Too often, the emphasis in our programs is on students' competency in biomedical knowledge, technological proficiency, such as interpreting evidence displayed on a monitor to guide decision-making, and/or their psychomotor skills such as doing an intravenous insertion in clinical practice. Students need to learn that compassionate interactions are not only as important as these other skills but also different from other social interactions. Compassionate communication purposefully engages people and families to understand who they are and what matters to them, discern how they feel about their care experience, and together develop a plan of care (Dewar 2013). As educators, we must ask ourselves how we are teaching compassion. Are we holding on to the safety of our life preserver by using the pedagogies and knowledge we are most comfortable with? Are we using the traditional method of the "sage on the stage" with our slide deck on how to be compassionate, subjecting our students to "death by PowerPoint"?

Some people question whether compassionate care can be taught or it is an innate attribute that some have and others don't. In a recent study that we conducted with colleagues (Mallette, Rose, et al. 2018), students overwhelmingly described how their innate ability to care drew them to a healthcare profession. Yet one student expressed concern that the capacity to care is a "personality trait that is developed before starting the program ... If there is no seed in the ground, you are just watering dirt and nothing will grow." Each person has their own ability to provide care and their own understanding of compassion, shaped by their cultural backgrounds, social environments, and past interactions with others. The purpose of providing education related to compassion is to foster and develop each student's awareness of their own innate ability that they can then apply in their professional roles. As educators we must also grapple with the dilemma that if future healthcare professionals will require different knowledge and skill sets with compassionate care as one of them, should we embrace those applicants who have an overall A+ GPA, yet do not have the *seed to grow* – the inability to be compassionate?

Reflective practices have been identified as a key learning strategy to assist students' development of compassionate care practices and are often a critical component of curricula within health professional education programs (Landy, Cameron, et al. 2016, Nguyen, Fernandez, et al. 2014). These practices are not about teaching students how to be kind or how to think and feel. Instead, reflective practices build students' awareness of their own identities, past experiences, and positioning within larger social contexts, as these all influence their ability to be compassionate (Song and Stewart 2012). Reflective practices need to be used throughout educational programs to support students' growth and development in providing compassionate care. In this way, students will view reflective practice not as something irrelevant, only to be done in their program's first semester but rather as something that should occur over the course of their professional careers (Song and Stewart 2012).

We must also examine what we emphasize, and when, in our students' learning. Is the focus on biomedical knowledge and/or technological and psychomotor tasks, or do we also focus on how to provide compassionate care while applying this knowledge and performing these tasks? Taran (2015) highlights that educational programs are not reinforcing the importance of the ability to provide compassionate care. As a result, students can view lectures on these topics as a time to catch up on social media and sleep or not attend the lecture.

Within the academic environment, theories and practices of compassionate care are usually taught in the first semester of health professional programs using reflective practices and experiential learning strategies, such as arts-based learning, simulation, and case studies. However, following the first year of these programs, the focus usually shifts to biomedical knowledge and technological and psychomotor skills for the rest of the students' education. As an unintended consequence, these can be viewed as the most valuable forms of knowledge and skill in both the academic and clinical environments. Compassionate care can become lost or viewed as secondary.

Within health professional programs, compassionate care concepts should be interwoven throughout the program rather than relegated to the first semester. The knowledge, skills, and attitudes related to compassionate care learned in the first year should be considered as building blocks for future learning (Brown 2011). At the novice level, the objectives could focus on the student's awareness of the concepts. At more advanced levels, students should become accountable for providing compassionate care while implementing their knowledge and skills (Brown 2011). An example of this could be learning how to participate in a cardiac arrest. As a novice, students might be expected to focus on the technological and psychomotor skills needed for resuscitating the person. As they become proficient in these skills, they should then also be expected to provide compassionate care to the person and their family.

Michelle's Reflection

The importance of this ability comes to life with an experience I had walking through a large urban emergency ward. As I waited to meet a colleague, I noticed a woman sitting just down the hall. Whatever was happening behind the trauma room door, she was part of it. She was visibly upset, crying, "I wonder if he knows I am here ... No one is saying anything, and all those people are in there." Once in a while, the door would swing open, and a person in scrubs would come out with a pager in one hand, phone in the other, moving past her and never once looking her way. The door would swing open and the world would open up. There were teams working in that room. A team leader with an iPad in hand called out orders without looking up. Another person was recording, not looking up. Someone was doing compressions – a code, her child? I wondered what this woman would be left with. The fear that her child did not know she was there. She may as well have been on the other side of the world.

What are we doing? Even in a trauma room, in the midst of a code, we can find a safe space for a parent and compassionate care. I know this. I have been the nurse who stood behind a parent sitting on a rolling stool in the midst of an arrest, whispering into her child's ear, "I am here. Mommy is here." But we have to see beyond the dashboard of our iPad algorithms, electronic records, and tasks at hand. We have to return to our breath, to appreciate the tenuous thread between child and parent and "the passing" between this world and the next.

Returning to Caputo's reflection, we as educators need to prepare our students for the future and the unforeseeable. As we reflect on how to do this, the story comes to mind of Dorothy Vaughan's ability to prepare for the unforeseeable, depicted in the book and movie of the same title *Hidden Figures* comes to mind. Hodges (2018) describes how Vaughan recognizes that with the arrival of a machine called IBM, her role and the people who work with her, would become obsolete. Instead of standing on the shore of uncertainty and waiting for their jobs to become redundant, she jumps into the uncertainty by reading the operating manual and training herself and her colleagues to become computer programmers.

As educators, we must prepare our students for new roles and ways of practicing rather than becoming redundant. No longer will our students have to memorize and retain all the information necessary to care for their patients. Our current curricula, largely based on memorization, will need to be reoriented toward ensuring that future health professionals have the competence to effectively, responsibly, and compassionately integrate and use the vast amount of available information in their practice (Wartman and Combs 2018). They will need to become curious practitioners. Curiosity motivates learning through a willingness to extend knowledge and become comfortable with uncertainty (Hartrick Doane and Varcoe 2015). Being curious means that knowledge, values, thoughts, emotions, actions, and practices can all be questioned and explored to find other ways to provide professional practice and compassionate care.

Our future curious practitioners will need to be prepared to use big data and technology appropriately with a critical lens. Critical thinking to explore what is appropriate for each person's circumstances and experiences will also be essential to students' practice. Otherwise, students will be at risk of developing a false sense of security in recommended and standardized plans of care regardless of individual experiences and a person's desire for inclusion in the decision-making process. Critical thinking in educational programs will also be necessary to ensure that students develop the capacity to access, analyze, and synthesize vast amounts of information to make clinical and population-based decisions in compassionate and equitable ways. As future healthcare practitioners, they will be part of global networks while participating in patient- and population-centred health systems. They will need to engage in critical reasoning and ethical conduct both within local health systems and within globally connected teams (Frenk, Chen, et al. 2010).

As teachers, we will need to shift our focus from *what* we teach to *how* we teach (Kahn, Maurer, et al. 2014). Practice will also be guided through collective intelligence, complementary ideas, and creativity (Bruce 2018; Frenk, Chen, et al. 2010). To develop students' ability to master large amounts of information in finding the most appropriate solutions, teaching practices should encourage active, creative, and collaborative learning (Bruce 2018; Frenk, Chen, et al. 2010). We will need to embrace the tools our students are familiar with while guiding them in the importance of humanism in providing compassionate care.

An example of this balance is a change initiative assignment that was created in a nursing leadership course for undergraduate students at York University in Toronto, Ontario. As educators, we often rely on traditional assignments and evaluation methods, such as group presentations to the class. For this course, one of the evaluation measures was changed to recognize the value of – and students' preference for – a variety of learning experiences. The purpose of the assignment was to impress upon students the power they have as change agents.

The challenge was to engage the students in forging human connections (processes we are familiar with) while embracing the mediums students were comfortable using to convey their ideas and messages: students were required to implement a change initiative with the use of social media strategies. The assignment was based on the Change Day initiative, launched in Ontario by Associated Medical Services and Health Quality Ontario. The initiative challenges participants to effect change by taking actions, large or small, to collectively improve the healthcare system. Individual acts of change, regardless of their extent, can add up to significant improvements for Ontarians, the profession, and the healthcare system overall.

At the beginning of the semester, students self-selected into groups to explore and critically analyze an issue related to nursing that they were passionate about. They were then required to implement a change initiative to address the issue through creating a social media strategy. To carry out this assignment, the students needed to talk with people to better understand the issue and to create their change initiative (fostering the human connection), and then convey what they learned through familiar mediums, such as Facebook, Instagram, and Twitter. Their initiatives explored important issues in healthcare such as bullying, the opioid crisis, inequities in healthcare in Northern Ontario, mental health, and political action. Their sites had multiple views (most over 100 and for some over 1,000) and followers. The students loved doing the assignment.

> Claire's Reflection
> Through this assignment, both the students and I learned about the power of social media in creating change. I also realized the importance of tapping into the students' expertise in using technology to make a difference in ways that I could never have imagined, while ensuring that they continued to learn the importance of the human connection.

We also have to acknowledge how pervasive social media has become within society and healthcare. As educators, we need to understand how students can leverage social media in relation to their professional education. We need to be asking what uses are appropriate and how these questions should be incorporated into our curricula.

In teaching our students, we can embrace social media as a learning tool: a way to promote communication among and between students and faculty, to build professional networks, and to learn new communication skills to employ with patients (Arrigoni, Alvaro, et al. 2016). Social media can be very beneficial for conveying health information to patients and connecting them with appropriate resources and communities of support. However, students need to become cognizant of the difference between social and professional communication in these forums since there can be a fine line between proper and improper use (Arrigoni, Alvaro, et al. 2016). Students also need to learn the importance of privacy and how not to breech confidentiality when using social media to communicate with and about their patients.

Another area of concern that causes turbulence between educators and students is the sense of anonymity when communicating through a screen. Students may feel able to speak freely without the filter of social norms that exists when communicating face to face. Each of our healthcare professions and educational programs has policies outlining appropriate communication on social media. Yet, all of us have experienced students posting inappropriate comments on the internet (some under the guise of a private chat room, which isn't really private), including information about their patients and opinions about classmates, practitioners, or professors. When approached to discuss their behaviour, students will often claim that their online comments do not reflect their true behaviour as a person. This situation highlights the difference between us as educators who learned how to communicate with very different social boundaries and our students who use a screen as the primary mode of communication. The challenge lies in recognizing that our students are still learning the nuances of professional communication and its boundaries versus social interactions. Those nuances are further complicated by social media technologies, which have made boundaries between professional, personal, and public spheres far more porous and ambiguous than ever before. Our experiences can help students to understand what it means to communicate therapeutically and professionally, face to face. We need new teaching strategies to consider, together, how these traditional norms and practices relate to communication practices in other media, including those that provide an apparent safety net of anonymity.

As we three ponder how our educator role is changing and how we can embrace technology in our teaching and learning strategies, we notice that our students have left our space and are swimming toward the space of possibilities and turbulence within the practice setting.

TURBULENCE IN THE PRACTICE SETTING

Learning how to become a compassionate health professional comes to life in the clinical environment. Activities in the academic environment, such as reflective exercises, role playing, and simulation, help students become more aware of their own values and beliefs and more comfortable in providing compassionate care. However, it is when students apply their knowledge in the practice environment that they begin to recognize the responsibility of caring for an actual patient. As one student in our study said, "It's not until you're at the bedside … that you actually realize that you are caring for a person, not just the simulation doll or a wound or a broken arm." Another stated, "They can teach you all you want about therapeutic communication and compassion, but you have to go into a clinical setting to really practice it and see what it means." (Mallette, Rose, et al. 2018, 28).

As students continue within the practice environment, they begin to feel turbulence in trying to implement what they have learned in the academic environment because the expectations in practice settings are very different. Some students are asked why they would ever want to become a health professional in the present healthcare environment. Others are told that "everything you have learned in school will mean nothing in practice." Students also discover that great emphasis is placed on their competence in performing technical skills in a timely manner. They begin to learn that technical efficiency is what matters most in the practice environment and is what they are judged on. Sadly, this often results in leaving compassionate care on the shoreline, as it is not a priority.

Clinical educators and practitioners are integral to students' learning as they facilitate students' application of the theories and knowledge they acquire. Positive clinical role models and educators are imperative to teaching students that the focus should not only be on competence in technical skills. These clinical teachers also need to focus on how students perform procedures while supporting the patients compassionately. To do this, educators in both academic and clinical environments need to recognize the novice-to-expert learning continuum. Novice learners can only concentrate on the procedure that needs to be performed. However, as they move toward competence in this area, the expectations, feedback, and evaluation of students' performance should include the integration of compassion along with knowledge and technical competence in meeting the needs of patients and families (Benner 1984). One student expressed this by asking, "What if they evaluated how you can communicate with your patient while you are going through this dressing change? I've never had a comment about that … [N]ever have they ever said, you didn't talk to your patient, see if they are okay, do they have pain, and you need to do this." (Mallette, Rose, et al. 2018, 34).

Clinical educators and practitioners also need to help students incorporate compassionate care into their practice amid the challenges of present work environments. Workloads are increasing, as are pressures to do more in less time. Educators need to teach and to role model how compassionate care can be achieved, even though professional practice is usually done "on the move," leaving little time to sit with a patient (Hartrick Doane and Varcoe 2015). Students and health professionals often believe they do not have time to develop relationships and to relate compassionately with patients and families. As educators, we need to emphasize that with every interaction students are in fact relating with the patient and family. What matters is how they "choose" to relate with them (Hartrick Doane and Varcoe 2015). Herbst, Swengros, and Kinney (2010) describe the "spinning" nurse who moves quickly and does more in less time by completing one task while anticipating the next. For example, while physically completing a dressing change, the nurse is already thinking of what medications are due. In this scenario, the nurse is choosing to focus only on the tasks rather than relating compassionately with the patient while doing the dressing change.

Another example would be the student or professional who chooses to look at the computer or iPad screen instead of looking at the patient. This has been described as "screen-side" manner rather than "bedside' manner," leading to more distant and impersonal interactions with patients. In this scenario, the student or professional is choosing to give all their attention to the screen instead of the person they are with. In some ways, this could be perceived as easier and more efficient, since the computer does not ask difficult questions – such as, "Please tell me, am I dying?" – which may leave the professional at a loss for an answer, concerned about time, and/or fearful of the patient's response.

When providing care, the student will need to choose whether to focus on the technology or use the technology to assist in providing humanistic, compassionate care. Educators need to assist students in recognizing when they are "spinning" and/or avoiding difficult conversations in order to refocus on being in the moment with the patient. This can be achieved through reflective practices, case studies, simulations, and positive role modelling in academic and clinical environments. Through these types of educational activities, students can learn that practices as simple as turning the computer screen toward patients can convey compassion. As students continue down the river in the space of possibilities created within practice settings, they notice practitioners who, while still swimming, seem to be flailing in the water and are at risk of going under. The students quickly swim to shore to retrieve some life preservers, fortuitously placed there, and help the practitioners don them. Once the practitioners are no longer at risk of drowning, they begin to tell stories of how the system prevents them from providing compassionate care for their patients in the ways they want to. The students listen attentively to the practitioners' concerns about workplace cultures in which the promotion of productivity, efficiency, and effectiveness can lead to a production-line mentality, with standardized care maps and frequent references to the "turnover" and "processing" of patients (Crawford, Brown, et al. 2014; Dewar, Loong, et al. 2014). While compassionate care is valued within organizations, the emphasis is primarily on standardized technical, clinical, and administrative policies and procedures. The practitioners share that they are burnt out and worried about their own health in trying to do their best to deliver compassionate care for their patients while meeting these multiple demands. They yearn for the compassionate organizations described in chapter 7 of this book, which prioritize compassion alongside efficiency. Some practitioners say that if the system does not change, they are contemplating swimming to shore and getting out of the river, leaving their profession.

While the practitioners tell their stories, the students begin to reflect on their own feelings of burnout, which have begun to set in even before they are practicing health professionals. They find it difficult to manage the workload to succeed in the clinical environment alongside competing demands in the academic environment. They feel overwhelmed with assignments and examinations due at the same time as they prepare for their clinical experiences. Worrying about succeeding in course assignments prevents them from attending compassionately to patients and families in the clinical setting. This double workload burden can lead students to feel mentally and physically exhausted. One student described this as educational burnout, resulting in apathy. They remember their teachers advising them to develop resilience by eating healthy food, getting eight hours of sleep, exercising regularly, identifying activities that reduce stress, and incorporating those activities into their lifestyle. However, during their time together, their teachers didn't help them find realistic activities that would actually achieve resilience and self-care within environments not designed to support such efforts.

TURBULENCE OF CARING FOR THE PERSON

Feeling worried that they, too, will soon need a life preserver to keep going, and perplexed by what they have experienced within the practice setting, the students decide to swim toward us educators to learn more about how they can not only survive but thrive as curious, compassionate practitioners. As we listen to the students' stories, we remember our readings from Caputo, that to face the unforeseeable we might shore up one another, draw on one another's unique wisdom to navigate the unknown, and embrace turbulence in meaningful ways. Together, we can all learn how to best embrace advancing technology and the system issues in the present and the future, both foreseeable and unforeseeable. We then ask our students to help us swim to the practice setting space to continue our journey.

As we get closer to where the practitioners are swimming, we notice there is another group moving at different speeds downriver. Some are still strongly navigating the waters, while others are using their life preservers as support; behind them, there are people clutching onto their life preservers for dear life, hoping they are not about to go under. As we look carefully at them, we come to realize that this group needs our care.

The people we care for have different comfort levels in using and understanding the technologies they encounter. Some are very conversant within the technological world, embracing all that technology has to offer, and want to be active members of the healthcare team. These people will have used the internet to research their symptoms, their diagnosis, and the most current treatments and how to access them. They will also have looked at their own EMR (if available) and researched what their diagnostic results mean. In all likelihood, they will also have searched social media sites related to their health concerns to learn from others' experiences.

Others we care for may not be as computer proficient, but still may have used Dr Google to get an understanding of what their diagnosis means. Clutching onto those life preservers for support, they want to be active participants in their care but may not have the knowledge, ability, or access to approach it in a more informed way. As curious practitioners, we must be attuned to these discrepancies and adapt our care accordingly. We also must not assume that a patient's age predicts which type of swimmer they are. Just the other day, Claire's ninety-year-old mother reported reading about a "low salt level" known as hyponatremia, saying that Google had told her to follow up with her doctor.

Our informed patients change the relationship that we have with them. No longer can we believe that healthcare professionals hold all the knowledge. Patients can and will be informed on the type of healthcare they want to receive. Educators, students, and practitioners will have to shift their focus from primarily "doing" clinical tasks for patients to "being" in a partnership with them in managing their care. Their practices will need to incorporate meaningful forms of patient engagement and empowerment so that patients become truly active members of the healthcare team. To address this shift in practice, we educators will need to shift our attention from knowledge and skills to adaptability in highly complex, dynamic, and uncertain environments. As future practitioners, students will also need to learn how to work collaboratively with the patient, their family, and the healthcare team, using big data appropriately, effectively, and most importantly with compassion.

Both students and practicing health professionals will need to expand their assessments to learn about each patient's and family's knowledge level related to their particular health concerns, accessibility to information, digital literacy, and engagement in social media networks. This will enable the healthcare providers to work alongside patients and families, while minimizing risk related to misunderstanding or misinformation on the internet. In their assessments, they should also not assume that the people they care for have appropriate computer and digital access and literacy; while some will have access to health information and data, others will not.

TURBULENCE OF TECHNOLOGY

None of us – educators, practitioners, or the people in need of care – can move forward successfully alone in addressing the turbulence of technology in education and practice. One way technologies create turbulence is by changing the relationship between the practitioner and patient. Until now, these relationships focused on supporting the person and family by providing emotional, physical, and informational support, as well as advocating for and empowering both (Arnold and Boggs 2019; Richardson, Percy, and Hughes 2015). These relationships are now changing to include not only the practitioner, person, and family, but also technologies themselves. This last section considers sources of turbulence or uncertainty that stem from learning to engage with new, non-human, members of the healthcare team.

Working collaboratively with technology is more effective and creative than working alone or competing with the technology (Almerud, Alapack, et al. 2008; Barnard 2016; Associated Medical Services 2017). When technology works effectively, it can be an excellent resource in guiding safe and effective care outcomes for healthcare professionals (Barnard 2016). However, educators, students, and practitioners need to be cognizant that technology can reduce practice to measurable and predictable actions designed to adhere to guidelines and protocol-based care (Barnard 2016). Conflict may arise when patients and families want to participate in directing their own healthcare experience, while health professionals prefer to follow the efficient and effective plan of care derived from big data analysis and organizational policies and procedures (Barnard 2016). Our students will need to navigate these conflicts through learning how to use a critical lens to listen, see, question, and apply their knowledge in order to incorporate compassion into their practice while using the best that technology can offer.

As Hodges describes in the introduction to this book, healthcare professionals do their best work when they balance the technical and human dimensions of healthcare. But what role will technology play? Moving forward, the temptation to replace human roles with technology will persist. As educators, we will need to create curricula that integrate the understanding of how technology and practitioners work together. One should not exist without the other, although human beings should remain at the centre of the practitioner-patient-technology triad, with the health practitioner and patient deciding on the appropriate role for technology in the delivery of care.

As educators, we will need to also keep abreast of the capabilities and limits of advancing technology. Robot technology cannot yet completely replace humans in providing comprehensive care to patients. In *The Economist* article on robonurses, the authors highlight that Japan leads the world in advanced robotics ("Pepper-Uppers – Japan is Embracing Nursing Care Robots," 2017). They are developing "carerobos" for their elderly population to address the increasing shortage of human care providers. They describe how robots presently do not have "sontaku," the ability, for instance, to infer from looking at a person that they would like a cup of tea. Humans do. Caputo (2018, 265) acknowledges the following:

> In the present state of the art, computers can calculate strictly cognitive problems, but they run up against a wall, sometimes literally, when they hit hermeneutics. They reach their limits when they are required to interpret, that is, to do things that cannot be solved by calculation but only by negotiation. They are stumped when they encounter a novel situation where, unprepared by any rule, what is required is a fresh judgment. Robots are matchless in performing routinizable operations, whereas simple but unprogrammable things, like turning a doorknob, are just too tricky for them. As someone quipped, if you want to protect yourself against the Terminator, just close your door.

While this is the state of robotic technology today, it would be naïve of us educators to ignore the constant evolution of AI. Presently, our curricula recognize the importance of interprofessional and interdisciplinary collaborations. Yet, programs continue to be implemented for the most part in silos with minimal, if any, interactions. Future healthcare teams with multiple healthcare providers (e.g., nurses, physicians, social workers, healthcare assistants), patients, families, and social groups (in person and virtually through social media such as Facebook, blogs, and beyond) will demand that the silos be broken down, with more collaborative learning and practices occurring (Wartman and Combs 2018).

Educators, students, and healthcare professionals will need to inform the design, selection, and implementation of health technology advancements. If we do not do this, then the adage "if you are not at the dinner table, you might be on the menu" may come to pass, as many technology firms see the financial possibilities in developing robotics for healthcare. Our participation in the ongoing advancements is essential in ensuring patients' healthcare concerns are met in a compassionate way while incorporating the use of technology in a safe, efficient, effective, economical, and ethical manner (McCabe and Timmins 2016; Risling 2017).

To achieve this, our curricula will need to include dedicated informatics courses focusing on competency in using knowledge and information platforms and methods to inform technology advancement (Risling 2017; Wartman and Combs 2018). Relationships should also be nurtured through collaborative learning activities introduced into our curricula with students and faculty from professional programs, such as computer science, engineering, design, and business. This will enable dialogue across disciplines on the future of healthcare technologies even before students graduate.

While ethical practice is addressed in all of our health professional curricula, we now need to incorporate significant ethical issues that emerge with the introduction of AI and robotics. We will need to explore with our students the new moral choices they will encounter within the practitioner-patient-technology interface. A more robust and systematic ethical and moral dialogue is required to examine the different care values at stake in healthcare practices that embrace technology (van Wynsberghe 2013). If care values are typically understood contextually by human beings, then how does the technology-human interface transform our understanding of values important to the human condition, and what role does technology play in providing care to the person? As van Wynsberghe (2013) suggests, a robot providing the simple act of bathing a person is an example of providing hygiene, safety (water temperature), and proper positioning to prevent injury. But, when humans bathe someone, they understand that the task is far more complex than providing hygiene, safety, and positioning. There is also the interplay of values, privacy, communication, empathy, dignity, respect, and compassion.

As educators, we must heed van Wynsberghe's (2013) challenge to pay attention and address with our students how moments of *caring about* and *caring for* people are essentially about preserving and promoting values of compassion aimed at sustaining the well-being of the people in need of care. From this perspective, care moments are spaces where trust, humility, vulnerability, responsibilities, and obligations are lived out between the person and practitioner (Hartrick Doane and Varcoe 2015; van Wynsberghe 2013). Ultimately, care ethics from a technology perspective are not so much about applying a particular ethical framework but more about understanding the complex interface of practices, people, technologies, and contexts. How do these interfaces manifest moral elements, including attentiveness, responsibilities, competency, responsiveness, and compassion (van Wynsberghe 2013)?

Lastly, with advancing technology and the introduction of robotics into healthcare environments, curricula will have to adapt to the changing focus and roles of future health professionals. Increased emphasis will need to be placed on knowledge and skills in the areas of complex interactions that care robots and technology cannot perform. This includes knowledge and skills in communication, assessments, critical thinking, collaborating, navigating, and negotiating, while developing the humanistic qualities of compassionate care such as empathy, values promotion, dignity, and trust. Emphasis will need to increase on social determinants of health, equity, ethics diversity, and health promotion (Bruce 2018; Risling 2017; van Wynsberghe 2013).

ARRIVING AT A NEW SHORE

We continue to navigate downriver, supporting and learning from one another, contemplating the awareness we have gained by encountering different tensions and spaces of possibility. We then see a new shore that beckons us to step out of the river and begin applying what we have learned. While technologies will continue to change, we have found new footing in our educational and clinical practices. As educators, we may use new media and methods to educate our students and provide care, but the need for human connection will always persist – this is what we must strive to pass on to our future curious, compassionate practitioners.

We educators begin to discuss what is necessary to advance our curricula. One of us suggests telemedicine as an example of what is the future needs. Presently, telemedicine is a virtual space for conducting healthcare encounters to diagnose, monitor, provide treatment, and offer education and support systems. It is often used where there is limited access to health services, such as in rural and remote areas. Telemedicine technologies will continue to grow and develop, with more people accessing healthcare providers from wherever they are, instead of expending time and money travelling to hospitals or sitting in an office waiting for a healthcare appointment. The location and form of future healthcare interactions are only limited by our imaginations. Preserving the human connection in these interactions will be imperative.

Michelle's Reflection

I was involved in conducting research exploring the educational competencies that practitioners will need when doing video oncology appointments. I remember a telemedicine nurse describing what it is like to be
in the room with a patient who is seeing a specialist via video in a large
urban hospital. She started by describing the sorts of technological skills
required: how to position a camera to zoom in on a wound, or how
to position a stethoscope and adjust the sound to capture value clicks.
She emphasized the need to be skilled with physical assessment at an
advanced level, as you are the eyes and ears of a specialist. But what
stuck out in my mind was her fleeting comment about the "little things
you do – you know, the nursing things." Nursing things, like being
another set of eyes and ears to capture what the specialist says, and how
at times a practitioner's presence brings comfort. She recalled helping
a patient with complications from radiation therapy, and how, out of
sight of the camera, the person gripped her arm so tightly with fingers
digging into her skin, afraid that the skin reaction meant the cancer had
progressed. This was something that the technology would not have
captured without the presence of a human being. Later, when we asked
patients and families about their experiences of video telehealth, they
emphasized "familiar support": the presence of nurses and other care
providers who were familiar with them and their condition, who had
the ability to step in and advocate for their needs. (Sevean, Dampier,
et al. 2008)

This reflection gives us pause in examining how to move forward
to ensure the human connection, compassion, and the "familiar support" are not lost in our curricula of the unforeseeable. As educators,
we are the first ones to guide, teach, and influence our future practitioners. We have the responsibility of ensuring they have the knowledge and skills to be curious, compassionate practitioners in this new
technological world.

We reflect on where we began this journey, and the teachings of
Caputo resonate once again. We remember that only through intention, attention, and working together can we better see what lies ahead
to prepare ourselves and our students for the unforeseen future. We
realize that we cannot stay safe on the shores of the status quo being
reactive in our curricula to the changes in healthcare. Too often, we
are the last ones to jump into the river of possibilities, and if we do

jump in, we are holding on to the life preserver of our old ways of knowing and teaching. Instead, we must be proactive, showing leadership in preparing our students for the future by being the first ones not simply entering the river but diving in.

The words of Antoine de Saint-Exupéry bear repeating: "It is the compelling zest of high adventure and of victory, and in creative action, that man finds his supreme joys" (de Saint-Exupéry 1950, 86). During the time together with our students, we have the responsibility not only to inculcate the importance of compassion within the technological world of healthcare but also to show how it can be incorporated into their practice. We need to provide them with the necessary knowledge and skills to prepare them for being nimble in providing curious, compassionate care while adapting to advancing technology. We must also ensure that we assist our students in finding their courage, which will enable them to practice compassionate care regardless of the turbulence around them. We need to become the Dorothy Vaughan of health education to enable our students to confidently navigate the turbulence of the unforeseen. Thus, instead of remaining on the shore of status quo, our students swim strongly through turbulence with the "zest of high adventure." They achieve a sense of victory and joy in making a difference. They apply their knowledge and skills not as robots do but with the creative action that only humans can provide. These are the qualities of curious, compassionate practitioners who will be able to meet the needs of the people they care for within the unforeseeable healthcare of the future.

6

Compassionate Leadership

*Maria Tassone, Jill Shaver, Mandy Lowe,
Catherine Creede, and Kathryn Parker*

A STORY OF COMPASSIONATE
LEADERSHIP IN ACTION[1]

This story begins in an urban academic hospital network at a time when the organization had begun implementing an Advance Care Planning (ACP) initiative. Many professionals across the organization were being asked to initiate conversations with patients about their values, beliefs, and preferences regarding treatment and care. Patients were encouraged to identify people whom they would trust to act upon their wishes if they became unable to make or to communicate their own decisions.

As this initiative was implemented across the organization, stories of discomfort began to surface. Many healthcare providers felt that they did not have enough knowledge, expertise, and support to enable patients to articulate what they did and did not want regarding their care. Enabling patients to share their wishes required individual care providers, leaders, teams, and the organization to attend to, understand, empathize with, and help address this area of unmet need and distress for all involved.

Noticing that many stories were surfacing organically, a small group of leaders created a video montage featuring care providers, leaders, and patients illustrating the importance of ACP. The video of first-person stories acted as a catalyst and seemed to give permission for many others to share their stories. The need to better address ACP became more compelling, setting the stage for the next phase of work. The same small group of leaders began this next phase by defining the purpose or intention of the ACP initiative. During this work, they realized that they themselves had not had conversations about their own wishes with their loved ones; few had articulated their own advance care plan. By initiating these conversations themselves, the leaders developed a deeper understanding of the challenges inherent to this process. They gained empathy for care providers, patients, and families, along with insights about how to support them through these difficult conversations. This experience with their own loved ones also shifted how the leaders thought and talked about this work. They began using more personal language to describe the purpose of the initiative. For example, talk of "substitute decision-makers" and a sense that "we know best" were replaced with a language of partnership and sense of shared human experience.

The leaders set out to learn more about what was already happening in the organization with respect to ACP. They began with structured questions. They wanted to know how the ACP initiative aligned with other priorities. What issues did people feel were important? What advice did they have to share about improving engagement with the ACP initiative? What did they need to support their leadership on behalf of this initiative? Although these kinds of questions had been used effectively with other initiatives in the organization, they sometimes elicited defensive and fearful responses when applied to ACP. "Why are you asking?" some people wanted to know. "What do I have to do?" People critiqued the initiative as too big. "You have bitten off more than you can chew."

It became clear that a new approach was needed. The imperative of ACP was striking a deep chord. The team co-created a new strategy for initiating meaningful conversations with care providers. It involved being completely present as an equal, with one prepared question, and no script, to explore a shared human experience. Each conversation began with the sharing of anonymized stories from patients, families, and care providers, and then one question was asked: "What has been *your* experience so far with ACP?" Follow-up questions emerged from a place of openness, curiosity, non-judgment, humility, empathy; a deep listening to the responses; and a sensing of what might remain to be said or shared. This approach yielded meaningful stories and suggestions, and people felt heard, respected, and valued.

This example illustrates a compassionate approach to leadership: an approach that grows from meaningful human connections and responds to human needs within complex organizations. In this chapter, we will describe the "being" and "doing" of compassionate leadership. We argue that this approach to leadership can help healthcare organizations remain aligned with their central purpose – providing compassionate care – especially in times of uncertainty when change is driven by multiple forces, including technologies with evolving, and sometimes threatening, human effects.

WHY COMPASSIONATE LEADERSHIP NOW?

Emerging technologies are expected to change healthcare more dramatically than they have in the past. As Marshall Goldsmith says, "What got you here won't get you there" (Goldsmith and Reiter 2007). Leadership for the future will need to be different. Compassionate leadership will be essential to navigating unprecedented changes in healthcare work as roles emerge, disappear, and become transformed by technologies. These changes are not just about implementing new tools.

At its heart, compassionate leadership concerns how we treat people – all people: how we notice, understand, empathize with, and help each other and ourselves as human beings. The compelling need for compassionate leadership has been well argued in recent literature, not only for today's healthcare organizations, but for all of us who either access life-saving and life-enhancing services or work within these organizations to provide them (Bottomley and Tehan 2006; de Zulueta 2016; Dutton, Workman, and Hardin 2014; West and Chowla 2017; West, Eckert, et al. 2017; Worline and Dutton 2017). Compassionate leadership, while often aligned with healthcare, is equally applicable to a wide range of contexts (e.g., administration, education, research, business). Perhaps surprisingly, compassionate leadership in healthcare has not been fully defined or conceptualized. It is most predominantly rooted in the idea of relieving suffering of patients (and, to a lesser extent, employees), and could benefit from a more expansive definition and approach.

Continuous technological advances in healthcare delivery demand a heightened awareness of how caring can be sustained through human interaction, particularly in highly demanding work environments. As more technology is integrated into healthcare, we need to be even more mindful about its potential effects upon our ability to be present, empathetic, and compassionate. For example, when procuring new technologies (e.g., electronic patient records), leaders must pay attention to who is affected and which voices inform decisions about products and their implementation. Decisions made must also preserve the centrality of compassion in healthcare.

Ultimately, compassionate leadership is directed toward patients, who are the primary focus of healthcare efforts; however, the need to create a culture to empower and support those who work in healthcare cannot be understated. In this way, compassionate leadership also becomes a primary strategy for addressing issues of burnout, compassion fatigue and satisfaction, and resilience that are so prevalent in healthcare organizations today. Leadership is seen as the most influential factor in shaping an organizational culture of compassion (de Zulueta 2016). When healthcare workers experience compassion and a compassionate work environment, they are more able and inspired to be compassionate toward the patients they serve, the various teams to which they belong, and their organization.

Compassionate leadership can also bolster quality of care in a variety of ways. It sets the stage for innovation among individuals, teams, and organizations as a whole (West, Eckert, et al. 2017; Worline and Dutton 2017), which will be essential for effective and sustainable implementation of new technologies. Compassionate leadership is necessary for an environment where people feel encouraged and safe to innovate (West, Eckert, et al. 2017). Compassionate leadership enables outcomes related to clinical effectiveness, patient safety, patient experience, efficiency, and staff engagement and well-being (West, Eckert, et al. 2017). It is also enables patients and their families to safely engage with the healthcare system when they are at their most vulnerable and to "have their humanity and uniqueness acknowledged" (de Zulueta 2016, 2). Compassionate leadership within healthcare therefore serves patients, healthcare workers, and the system at large.

Together with other leaders, several of us began exploring leadership twelve years ago as a small collective working in the health system in Ontario to develop a model of shared leadership that would help advance interprofessional practice. We co-created a model of Collaborative Change Leadership (CCL) that required practitioners, educators, and leaders to deeply consider the perspectives, lived experience, and knowledge of colleagues. This model is rooted in the principle that meaningful collaboration requires us to truly understand and value each other as human beings.

Over the past decade, through our CCL program, we have worked with approximately 200 healthcare and education leaders to develop their capacity for sustainable, empowering change leadership. Over that time, in collaboration with learners, we noticed a significant shift in many leaders toward a socially accountable and compassionate way of leading: one that was primarily situated in deep listening, honouring of diverse people and perspectives, and co-creating change that contributes to quality outcomes. To create an environment where patients are ensured high-quality, compassionate care, we need leaders who can create a compassionate work environment (de Zulueta 2016). Our belief is that CCL is the most effective way for compassionate leaders to lead change.

Building upon existing leadership theories, including CCL, this chapter advances a model of, and practices for, compassionate leadership. This model requires self-compassion, understands leadership as a state of being, integrates being with doing, and recognizes compassion as generative. We will provide a brief review of key leadership theories linked to compassionate leadership. We then present a framework that can be used to build the capacity of anyone at any point in healthcare to lead compassionately from where they are, no matter their current role or sphere of influence. We build on the ACP story to animate the core elements of compassionate leadership, for leadership at the individual, team, and organization levels. We end the chapter with considerations for cultivating compassionate leadership, especially for leaders in more formal leadership roles who are well positioned to create and influence a culture in which healthcare workers can be at their best and thrive in their day-to-day work.

LEADERSHIP THEORIES AND MODELS

There is a growing recognition that care must be both scientific and compassionate for the best patient outcomes. However, compassionate leadership remains poorly conceptualized within healthcare. Literature from the nursing profession describes compassionate leadership but does not articulate a theory, model, or framework (Ali and Terry 2017; Foster 2017; Hornett 2012; Turkel 2014). To advance such a model, we sought to build from our own work on collaborative change, along with a selective review of relevant leadership theories and models developed in other workplaces.

An important premise about leadership generally is that all who work in healthcare can lead; leadership is not reserved for those with formal leadership roles. Leadership involves dynamic, non-linear, reciprocal processes and outcomes, available to everyone and not restricted to a formally designated person (de Zulueta 2016). From this perspective, the traditional triad of leader, followers, and influencers is abandoned (de Zulueta 2016), as is the still-dominant model of heroic leadership.

In writing this chapter, we chose to highlight leadership theories that focus on nurturing relationships between people. This is in sharp contrast to more traditional leadership theories of command and control, which suggest that optimal results are best achieved through regimented and standardized practices, often resulting in the dehumanizing of individuals. We also purposefully included theories that link leadership to being of service and supporting the growth of an individual, group, or organization. These include strengths-based theories that focus on creating positive change and moving a group or organization toward a desired future. In reviewing these theories, and drawing upon our own lived experiences, we have realized that a deep understanding of compassionate leadership requires a fusing of several leadership discourses, particularly those related to *servant leadership* and cclc, along with key elements of transformational leadership, authentic leadership, ethical leadership, empowering leadership, resonant leadership, and appreciative leadership.

SERVANT LEADERSHIP

In servant leadership, effective leaders are always working toward "nurturing the personal, professional, and spiritual growth of the other" (Van Dierendonck 2011, 1232). In addition, they continually consider the far-reaching implications of their work, including intuitively foreseeing outcomes of situations, and being effective stewards to serve the needs of others (Spears 1995).

Robert Greenleaf coined the term *servant leadership* in his seminal essay "The Servant as Leader" (Greenleaf 1970). Although the term has been interpreted in multiple ways by a variety of authors and scholars in the last half decade, core to servant leadership is the notion that the leader is a servant first. As such, it is the most dominant leadership discourse that intentionally positions a leader as genuinely attending to the needs of others before the needs of the organization. Servant leadership begins with the natural and intrinsic feeling that one wants to serve, and follows with a conscious choice or aspiration to lead. According to Spears (1995, 4), "servant-leadership is a long-term, transformational approach to life and work, in essence, a way of being that has the potential to create positive change throughout our society." Grounded in Greenleaf's work, Spears suggests the best tests of servant leadership, although perhaps impossible to measure in empirical terms, are its powerful social effects: "Do those served grow as persons? Do they, while being served, become healthier, wiser, freer, more autonomous, and more likely to become servants? And, what is the effect on the least privileged in society? Will they benefit, or at least not further be harmed?" (Spears 1995, 4).

A servant-leader is first among equals, holds the organization in trust as one of its stewards, and is motivated by something more important than the need for power. The inspiration to lead comes from a commitment to the growth of individual employees, an organization's sustainability, and a responsibility to one's community. "Power becomes a possibility to serve others and as such may even be considered a prerequisite for servant-leaders. Serving and leading become almost exchangeable. Being a servant allows a person to lead; being a leader implies a person serves" (Van Dierendonck 2011, 1231).

Upon considering Greenleaf's original writings, Spears (1995) identifies what he believes are ten critical characteristics of a servant-leader: listening (emphasizing the importance of communication and identifying the will of the people); empathy (understanding and accepting others); healing (helping to make whole); awareness (having a more integrated view of situations); persuasion (influencing others and building consensus); conceptualization (balancing short-term goals with a visionary lens of the possible future); foresight (using the intuitive mind to foresee situational outcomes); stewardship (holding something in trust and serving the needs of others); commitment to the growth of people (nurturing the personal, professional, and spiritual growth of others); and building community (identifying and implementing strategies for fostering community in the workplace) (Spears 1995, 4–5).

More recently, compassionate love was proposed as an underlying motivation or cornerstone of servant leadership. Van Dierendonck and Patterson (2015) describe it in part as acts of kindness that are intended for the follower's benefit, not for that of the leader. Beyond acts, there is an orientation of openness and receptivity to seeing followers as "hired hearts versus hired hands ... thereby valuing the other at a fundamental level" (Van Dierendonck and Patterson 2015, 121–2).

Servant leadership speaks beyond the moment and speaks to the humanity within us all. It offers an approach that matches current cultural and organizational contexts where both leaders and followers "must seek to do the right things [... and offer ...] real-world solutions that are based on moral and virtuous strengths" (Van Dierendonck and Patterson 2015, 128).

Servant leadership intentionally positions a leader as genuinely attending to the needs of others before the needs of the organization. From a stewardship point of view, the healthcare mission, however, is to attend both to others' needs and to those of the organization itself. It is worth noting that this service-to-others compass is also complicated, in healthcare, by the imperative to put patients first. Therefore, compassionate leadership in healthcare needs to also focus on the organization as it serves the needs of others, including continuously changing and improving to better meet patient and community needs.

COLLABORATIVE CHANGE LEADERSHIP

CCL is a healthcare-specific leadership model we evolved over a decade ago in response to the increased need for working across teams, disciplines, professions, organizations, and systems. This approach represents a shift from the lone hero concept to an inclusive, collaborative approach that enables leaders to draw on the strengths and wisdom of any person or collective. We initially developed CCL through the lens of non-hierarchical interprofessional practice, of being "about, from, and with each other" (WHO 2010), and quickly married these ideas to several other key concepts.

We first focused on how collaborative change leaders could fully connect with and draw upon the strengths of everyone in their team or work group. For this, we integrated the key elements of Appreciative Inquiry, which fundamentally holds that when people are fully engaged in imagining and exploring the kinds of possibilities that feel energizing, they have the wisdom and capacity to make changes toward their desired future. In this context, CCL focuses people on strengths and what is "life-giving" in an organization (i.e., the things they most value) and supports them in moving toward the changes that feel most "right" to them. This assumes that different things are needed in every group to create the desired change. The work of the leader is to help a group identify what those things are in their own environment and to feel fully empowered in advancing toward the desired future (Whitney, Trosten-Bloom, and Rader 2010).

We draw on Appreciative Inquiry both as a process for leading change and as a theoretical underpinning for all of our work. Our central premise is that everyone has the capacity to contribute in creative and powerful ways, and the job of leaders is to bring that capacity to life. Healthcare is a complex system. No one leader can know the whole system. Therefore, to address the questions and issues that we face in healthcare, leaders must continually sense what is emerging and listen to many perspectives. In CCL, we help people become comfortable with emergence (Holland 1998; Westley, Zimmerman, and Patton 2006). Emergence is about noticing, responding to, and learning from small changes in the system, treating evaluation more as learning than assessment. We work with the principles of developmental evaluation (Patton 2010) to provide a framework for this often challenging approach to tracking change and adapting action appropriately. We also help participants develop their capacity to pay attention to many sources of information in the system. Participants learn the concept of collective intelligence: the belief that enacting a new system is not about getting the one right answer, but about developing networks of engaged and trusting people guided by a common understanding of the current systems and a commitment to creating a new direction (Jaworski 2012).

As we are building capacity for the kind of fluid, generative leadership required in complex systems, we facilitate a transformative individual experience for the learners. Central to this aspect of CCL is the concept of an individual's interior condition or being, the place from which our actions originate (Scharmer 2007b, 7). Leaders must be aware of and pay attention to their deep beliefs and assumptions, and recognize that "the quality of attention and intention that the leader brings to any situation" is consequential (Scharmer 2007a, 1). Two leaders doing the exact same things outwardly, or using the same processes, will have different effects and outcomes depending on the quality of humanity they bring (Scharmer 2007a). Self-awareness, as the vehicle for tapping into this being of leadership, is therefore positioned as the core or central concept of CCL.

From the initial position of deep self-awareness, leaders develop transformative practices to mobilize the wisdom, energy, diverse perspectives, and actions of people across an organization as they collectively identify new possibilities and co-create a desired future. Some of the practices we use to build this deep understanding include identifying and working with individual strengths, engaging in continual reflection, and exercising mindfulness to pay greater attention in a particular way "on purpose, in the present moment and non-judgmentally" (Kabat-Zinn 2016, 1).

Over time, we realized that it was important to add an explicit understanding of social accountability into our approach to CCL. Whether a healthcare system is publicly or privately funded, there is an inherent social accountability to all acts of change. When people seek to change their environments or practices, they are always working toward some greater good – whether this is enhancing an individual patient's experience, improving access to and equity of care, or shoring up the financial sustainability of the public health system. Successful leaders are aware of the consequences of their actions and foster spaces where others can bring their full, most generative selves to create elegant solutions for complex questions. With this element of social accountability, there is significant alignment between the model of CCL and servant leadership.

SIMILARITIES, DISTINCTIONS, AND OTHER RELEVANT THEORIES

In both servant leadership and CCL, leaders take the same stances of compassion, openness, humility, curiosity and non-judgment for themselves and others. In both theories, leaders bring their self-awareness to any moment, they listen deeply to the needs and perspectives of others, and they build community from a place of social good. Where the two models differ significantly is in the orientation of the leader. As previously stated, servant-leaders focus first and foremost on the needs of others before the organization. Collaborative change leaders engage and honour all perspectives to constantly move the organization toward the goal of better serving the needs of others.

Our understanding of compassionate leadership is also informed by selected principles from six additional leadership theories that are most aligned with compassion: transformational, authentic, ethical, empowering, resonant, and appreciative. We will describe briefly how these principles enhance our conception of compassionate leadership.

Transformational leadership focuses on the individual leader: before one transforms any system, there must be a transformation of self. Transformation of self is a necessary precursor to system transformation, which often starts with a "disorienting dilemma" as described by Mezirow (1991).

Authentic leadership is about expressing one's true self, including being aware of one's own values, life experiences, and how one sees the world, while simultaneously acknowledging and integrating others' uniqueness.

Ethical leadership demonstrates normatively appropriate conduct through personal actions and interpersonal relationships. It promotes such conduct to followers through two-way communication, reinforcement, and decision-making.

Empowering leadership emphasizes employees' self-influence processes and actively encourages followers to lead themselves through self-direction and self-motivation.

Resonant leadership describes effective leaders as those who cultivate relationships that rest on truly knowing other people as full human beings, attuning to them, listening closely to their frustrations and joys, and caring about them deeply (Worline and Dutton 2017).

Appreciative leadership focuses on five elements: inquiry (which enables people to see and feel that the leader values them and their contributions), illumination (which grounds people in understanding how they can best contribute their full talents and passions), inclusion (which creates an individual and community sense of belonging), inspiration (which provides the opportunity for new directions and possibilities to emerge), and integrity (which instills the hope and expectation that people will give their best for the benefit of the whole, trusting that others will do the same) (Whitney, Trosten-Bloom, and Rader 2010).

A MODEL OF COMPASSIONATE LEADERSHIP

Compassionate leadership in the context of Canadian healthcare builds on previous understandings of empathy (a noticing of and emotional response to someone else's need) and compassion (acting in response to empathy) and draws on the concept of "nurturing the best in others" that is embedded in both servant leadership and CCL. Compassionate leadership focuses on both process and outcome. Compassionate leaders "[lead] with the head and the heart" (Ali and Terry 2017, 78) while building capacity for compassion in others, within teams, and across organizations. Compassionate leadership can be individual or collective, and it can be practised by anyone.

Building on our experience and the leadership theories outlined earlier, we have developed the following portrait of compassionate

Compassionate Leadership Model

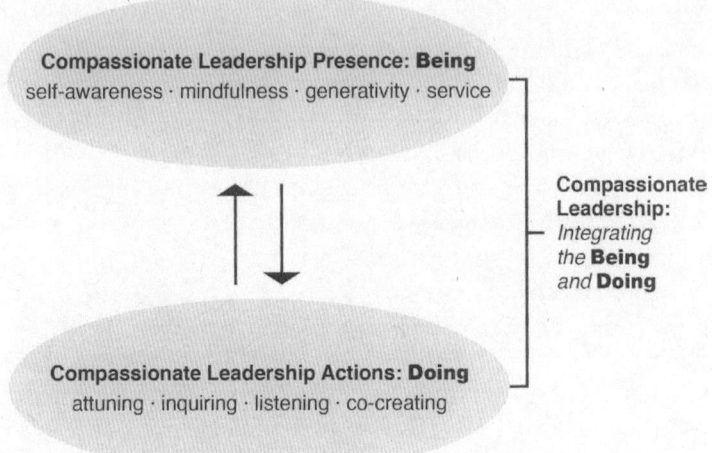

Figure 6.1 Compassionate leadership model

leadership for healthcare. As shown in figure 6.1, our compassionate leadership model, at a high level, encompasses compassionate
leadership presence (being) and compassionate leadership actions
(doing). The integration of being and doing is fundamental to
compassionate leadership.

COMPASSIONATE LEADERSHIP PRESENCE:
THE BEING OF COMPASSIONATE LEADERSHIP

Compassionate leadership is first about a way of being. The actions
of compassionate leaders are more powerful and effective when they
come from that state of being. Compassionate leadership is thus about
developing deep self-awareness, other-awareness, and compassion for
the purpose of optimizing the well-being of everyone, including ourselves. What we do flows from who we are as compassionate leaders.

Compassionate leadership presence addresses the essence of the
leader: the source from which the leader operates or acts. This presence encompasses four elements, which we will discuss in turn: self-
awareness, mindfulness, generativity, and service.

Self-Awareness

Self-awareness is at the core of compassionate leadership presence. It is the willingness to understand who we are, how we view ourselves, and how others experience us. With this insight and feedback, we realize where and how we can best serve as compassionate leaders. Our actions inform our self-awareness. This is depicted in figure 6.1 by the arrow flowing from compassionate leadership actions to compassionate leadership presence.

As leaders, our ability to articulate our own values and to understand that we are operating in a certain way based on those values is a precursor to being able to lead compassionately. Compassionate leaders are aware of their own values, how they live those values, and how they interpret the world, all while sensing and enabling the full humanity and potential of others.

Connected to this kind of self-awareness, our approach to compassionate leadership incorporates many of the principles of authentic leadership, which is focused on understanding our own motivations (Gardner, Avolio, et al. 2005) and acting in ways that are congruent with our deeply held values. In the most common definitions, authentic leaders are transparent, and their own ethical behaviour encourages openness in return (Gardner, Avolio, et al. 2005).

Practices to enhance the "being" of compassionate leadership are unique to each leader. Regardless of what the practices are, their value lies in their ability to deepen self-awareness through the letting go of judgment, cynicism, and fear, so that leaders can be "shockingly effective" (Jaworski 2012).

Mindfulness

The following eloquent description of mindfulness by Jon Kabat-Zinn (2016) deepens the presence, or being, of the compassionate leader. "Mindfulness is awareness, cultivated by paying attention in a sustained and particular way: on purpose, in the present moment, and non-judgmentally. It is one of many forms of meditation, if you think of meditation as any way in which we engage in (1) systematically regulating our attention and energy (2) thereby influencing and possibly transforming the quality of our experience (3) in the service of realizing the full range of our humanity and of

(4) relationships to others and the world." Mindfulness is particularly important amid all the noise and competing demands of complex healthcare organizations.

Generativity

The literature on compassion is largely problem-focused in that it is about the problem of pain and suffering and the fixing of the "problem" (i.e., alleviating the pain and suffering). This is often an appropriate focus for patient care, since there is usually pain and suffering of patients with respect to their medical condition and situation. However, little attention is paid to the unmet needs or, even more importantly, the full potential of individuals or organizations. Tending to others' suffering is necessary, but we must also attend to their full potential as humans. In chapter 2 of this collection, Rowland and Johannesen advocate for a similarly expansive approach to compassionate patient care and patient engagement. Creating a truly sustainable, thriving environment requires a broader definition of compassionate leadership that incorporates generativity.

Broadly defined, generativity is aimed at unleashing the most life-giving possibilities in any relationship or environment (Bushe 2012). Focusing compassionate leadership in a problem-based way establishes an inherently unequal relationship (e.g., one person is the sufferer, the other is the healer). We believe that the most powerful and generative relationships and innovation come when we treat each other as equals. If we choose a more generative approach to compassion, we acknowledge pain, suffering, and burnout, while also recognizing opportunities to draw upon their flip side, fostering resilience and finding meaning in work, hopes, and dreams. Specifically, it is important to understand when things are working well and how that is experienced, and then identify how to take action to bring the high point experiences into reality, each day, in every situation.

Our emphasis on generativity is strongly aligned with the "fourth aim" of finding meaning and joy in one's work, or cultivating clinician and team well-being and resilience, all prerequisites for sustainable healthcare. (This aim is often advocated as an expansion to Institute for Healthcare Improvement's "triple aim" of improving population health, enhancing patient experience, and reducing the cost of healthcare [Feeley 2017].) At its core, compassionate leadership is about incorporating the full humanity of everyone around you and enabling their unique potential and unnamed future.

Service

Compassionate leaders serve people. While many healthcare organizations are service oriented and prioritize the needs of patients first, our notion of service within the compassionate leadership model expands beyond this to include service to all: patients, families, healthcare providers, colleagues, learners, system partners, and ourselves.

While much of the literature on compassion and compassionate leadership has focused on being other-oriented, our model of compassionate leadership acknowledges our own presence and humanity. To be a compassionate leader, one also needs to have self-compassion (i.e., noticing one's own suffering and unmet needs, listening to oneself, understanding and empathizing with and helping oneself). One cannot have compassion for others without self-awareness or self-compassion. Leaders exercise self-compassion as they build their own capacity for compassionate leadership and aspire to be a compassionate leader all the time (i.e., have compassionate leadership as their operating system).

COMPASSIONATE LEADERSHIP ACTIONS: THE DOING OF COMPASSIONATE LEADERSHIP

Compassionate leadership actions flow from what we have described as the presence, source, or being of the leader. While any action can come from a place of compassion on the part of the leader, there are four specific actions within our Compassionate Leadership model: attuning, inquiring, listening, and co-creating.

Attuning

Attunement enables us to really know and understand another person by focusing on that individual's internal experience (including emotions, thoughts, and physiological experiences), from a place of curiosity, respect, and empathy. For example, a compassionate leader may focus on their breathing to help themselves become fully present to connect with the other person. When a leader takes action based on

attunement, there is resonance and the other person feels understood
and felt, which is essential for compassion (Boyatzis and McKee 2005).
In compassionate leadership, attuning is both the first and an ongoing
action: as leaders inquire, listen, and co-create, they continue to attune
to themselves and to the other(s).

Inquiring

Compassionate leaders inquire in order to understand and empathize
with the experience of others. Asking questions from a place of curiosity and humility enables others to share their emotions, thoughts,
and experiences. As authentic connections are made, generative questions are asked to begin to co-create the way forward, toward the fullest
possibility for an individual, a team, or an entire system. In essence,
our questions create our reality: words create worlds (Cooperrider
and Whitney 2005).

In the ACP story, for example, the team initially began their work
with questions that led to fearful and defensive responses. Based on
the answers, the team made an explicit choice, shifted to a more
generative stance, and asked questions that invoked meaningful stories
and suggestions. People felt heard, respected, and valued.

Examples of generative questions that could apply to a similar
context include: Reflect on and share a story of a special experience
when you enabled someone to share their ACP preferences. What
happened? What made that possible? What was the impact for that
person, for others, and for you? What are your hopes for how we
may all better enable patients to share their ACP preferences within
our organization?

Inquiring, as a powerful compassionate leadership action, is
insufficient without deep and vital listening.

Listening

Compassionate leaders listen with all of their senses for nuanced
information and new knowledge arising from individuals, teams, and
the collective. Bottomley and Tehan (2006) describe the importance
of vital listening, which is about listening deeply to others in a non-
judgmental way. This is done through narrative and storytelling and
supports the individual's sense of identity, self-worth, and belonging
(Bottomley and Tehan 2006). They also describe spacious listening,

an intervention that creates time and space needed for vital listening and affirmation of the essential truths of a respondent's experience. Through this type of listening, we place value on the choices and actions we take and identify any vulnerability, struggle, or need that is present. We also glean new insights into what support has already been marshalled, how effective it proves to be, and what other support may be needed.

This core element of listening is also enhanced by our understanding of psychological flexibility, defined as mindfulness and values-based action by Atkins and Parker (2012). Leaders who are more psychologically flexible are more sensitive to context, and therefore can better sense and listen for what particular actions are needed at any given time or in various environments.

Through vital and spacious listening with all of our senses, the foundation is laid for co-creating to alleviate suffering and address unmet needs.

Co-creating

In our model of compassionate leadership, we take the perspective that compassion is co-created. It is not enough to believe you are displaying empathy: you are not compassionate unless someone feels cared for. This co-creation is inherently reciprocal, and experiencing compassion makes people better able to show compassion to others (de Zulueta 2016). Compassionate leadership enables everyone in the system to bring forth their best to care for patients, each other, and the system's resources.

Compassion is inherently an emergent pattern; it emerges in individual conversations and in the collective, expanding far beyond a centralized approach (Worline and Dutton 2017). Leaders must be comfortable supporting emergent processes and practices that are not necessarily centrally identified and developed. Setting up team or organizational practices directed at compassion is about engaging with different stakeholders in the system.

Co-creating is also about how we engage with others to explore, design, and implement new possibilities and the changes necessary to alleviate suffering and address unmet needs (e.g., organizational structure, new scheduling system, patient care process, patient delivery models). In our ACP story, for example, the leaders with accountability for enacting ACP within the organization co-created the new way with patients, families, and healthcare providers. Through this continuous engagement, individuals who initially opposed what was being done joined the collaborative work and became part of the team moving it forward.

INTEGRATING THE BEING AND
DOING OF COMPASSIONATE LEADERSHIP

Literature on compassionate leadership has predominantly focused on what leaders *do*, especially on the behaviours of individuals in one-to-one interactions (Atkins and Parker 2012; West, Eckert, et al. 2017; West and Chowla 2017). Worline and Dutton (2017) went beyond the individual level and behavioural frame to integrate system-level concepts into their thinking about compassionate leadership (but not situated in healthcare). They position leaders, both formal and informal, as "social architects" of compassion within a system. This "leading for compassion" entails legitimizing suffering and compassion in an organization, using communication channels to reach a broad audience as a way of reinforcing a culture of shared humanity, and framing compassion as an emergent process versus a centralized approach.

These authors primarily focus on the doing of leadership – the acts, practices, or skills that translate into recognizable behaviours – yet, they miss the criticality of the "being" of leadership. As an example, imagine that you are meeting with a colleague and quickly notice there is something not quite right. During your discussion, he opens up and shares his concerns an issue that is troubling him. You are fully present as he discusses the challenges he is facing. You not only understand but also are able to fully empathize with him and offer several ways of helping. Afterwards, he tells you how truly grateful he is. He tells you that another leader had offered similar suggestions, but it felt to him like she was just trying to say the right things, like she was going through the motions of offering help. This is an example of the difference between the actions, or doing, that can be associated with compassionate leadership in contrast to the being of a compassionate leader. True compassionate leadership is felt by the other as the difference between feeling "treated" versus feeling cared for as a human being.

In our experience with the ACP initiative, one leader described the work as concerned with compassion, empathy, and being an equal in this human experience. They realized that to *do* this important work, they needed to *be* a compassionate leader: being an equal in (resonating with) the human experience and helping from a place of empathy. One of the leaders further realized that *being* without *doing* (helping or acting) is empathy, and *doing* without *being* is not necessarily compassionate. It risks being transactional and not felt by the other (a sense of being treated rather than being cared for).

The power of the compassionate leadership model is the inclusion of all eight elements (self-awareness, mindfulness, generativity, service, attuning, inquiring, listening, and co-creating), and more generally, the integration of presence and action. As previously described, leaders are "shockingly effective" (Jaworski 2012) when they are rooted in presence, or being. When a leader integrates and internalizes compassion in their being, and their doing is driven from their being, a leader practices and embodies compassionate leadership. When a leader is present and mindful, attuned to others, and connected to emerging needs, their compassionate actions will be meaningful.

Cultivating Compassionate Leadership

We have introduced a model of compassionate leadership and described what compassionate leaders do. Building on this foundation, we will now turn our focus to cultivating compassionate leadership at the level of self, dyad, team, and organization. Examples of practices that can be used to support compassionate leadership are listed in table 6.1.

Cultivating compassionate leadership begins at the level of self. To be a compassionate leader for others, one must first be a compassionate leader for self. For instance, in an airplane, we are told to put the air mask on ourselves first before putting it on anyone else. The practices focused at the level of self serve to integrate compassion into the leader's being. As compassion becomes more internalized and integrated, the being will be felt differently. In order for others to feel compassion from us, we must integrate being and doing to stay deeply present to what is emerging or needed in any situation.

Through one-to-one interactions and relationships, compassionate leadership expands from the self to include another person. In healthcare, cultivating compassion at the team level further expands compassionate leadership beyond the individual and the dyad. This has the potential of affecting everyone, including patients and healthcare

Table 6.1
Examples of practices for cultivating compassionate leadership

Levels of Focus	Practices
Self	• Observe and notice self • Practice mindfulness (e.g., be fully present in the moment, suspend judgment, notice your breath, meditate) • Journal • Practice yoga • Walk or spend time in nature • Reflect • Practice self-compassion • Be kind and gentle to yourself • Seek and integrate honest feedback from trusted individuals • Align internal and external states (be authentic)
Dyad (1:1)	• Build on the practices outlined at the level of self • Role model compassionate leadership • Be curious • Give and receive feedback • Coach each other • Discover strengths, meaningful similarities, and differences
Team	• Build on the practices outlined at the level of self and dyad • Create psychological safety • Conduct regular team check-ins (brief, focused personal sharing) • Create opportunities for shared leadership • Invite and share stories to foster understanding and connection • Create supportive space for sharing • Co-create statements of purpose and team charters • Honour the commitments we make as a team • Incorporate compassionate leadership actions in team charters and team interactions
Organization/ System	• Build on the practices outlined at the level of self, dyad, and team • Spread those practices across the organization and system • Incorporate compassion for all in the organization's values • Incorporate compassionate leadership in all organization processes, practices, and systems (e.g., hiring decisions and performance reviews) • Role model compassionate leadership at all levels of the organization • Track and evaluate the organization's compassionate leadership capability (e.g., employee survey, patient survey) • Celebrate and nurture compassionate leadership in others

providers. Furthermore, cultivating compassionate leadership as an organization can shift the organization's culture, which can ultimately have a ripple effect beyond the organization. Through cultivating compassionate leadership as individuals, teams, and organizations, compassionate leadership becomes integrated and embedded within healthcare.

During the ACP initiative, one of the leaders enhanced her awareness of her own suffering and unmet needs through self-noticing, understanding, and empathizing. Since her self-awareness manifested through her body (breathing, muscle tension) and her mind (inner dialogue), she helped herself by choosing to enhance her state of mindfulness (being fully present in the moment without judgment). She also practised helping behaviours related to self-compassion by exercising, meditating, focusing at the end of each day on how she has made a difference, savouring each moment, and practising being still (physically, emotionally, and cognitively), all as part of her preventative maintenance program.

At the dyad and team level, two leaders in our ACP story spoke about the importance of role modelling vulnerability to build capacity for compassion within the organization. When they shared their own personal experiences and feelings, it helped others access their emotions, empathy, and compassion that they had protected or hidden from others in the workplace.

In our ACP example, the organization's capacity for compassion was enhanced through specific practices, such as determining who was important to engage and how to engage, honouring and building on work that had already been done, inquiring, deeply listening, building on strengths, and co-creating.

As these practices become ingrained, they no longer need to be as consciously exercised, further enabling the compassionate leader to become fully present and self-aware. We can think about this as having some similarities to learning to drive. As we practised and learned to drive initially, we needed a remarkable degree of effort and coaching to attend to each step (checking mirrors, using the turn signal, etc.). However, as we became more proficient, these skills became more ingrained and automatic as we *became* drivers. We initially had to be intentional and methodical and pay attention, until it became automatic and we did not need to think about it; it just happened. We practice being a driver until we become, or are, one.

SUMMARY

Compassion for self and others will be critical as healthcare delivery is transformed with new technologies. As we adopt new ways of working, the leadership imperative is to ensure that compassion remains at the core of caring and healthcare. Compassionate leadership is a choice. It is also about building capacity for compassion that happens one person at a time. It is about patients, families, and all who work in healthcare feeling cared for. Leading for compassion involves communicating that we are all in it together and investing in the compassionate capacity of everyone. Leading for compassion may require significant transformational change in the policies, practices, and structures within an organization, but it starts from a place of "being" as a leader. As Carl Jung said, "Learn your theories as well as you can, but put them aside when you touch the miracle of the living soul" (Jung 1928, 361).

NOTE

1 We thank Daniela Bellicoso for her gracious assistance in the editing of this chapter.

Toward Compassionate Healthcare Organizations

Maria Athina (Tina) Martimianakis, Rabia Khan,
Erene Stergiopoulos, Marion Briggs, and Sandra Fisman

INTRODUCTION

"Staff inevitably catch up and adjust. What else can they do?"

Mark is an ambitious, charismatic leader who is passionate about rallying support for organizational changes that keep patients at the centre. He has very little tolerance for preventable medical errors and sloppy administration. Patients deserve better! There are so many new technologies that can help healthcare providers do their work more effectively and efficiently. Mark's goal is to improve wait times, reduce errors, increase workplace productivity, and decrease inefficiencies by revamping all hospital operations in the first five years of his term.

Technology is Mark's best friend. He knows the future of healthcare is in AI. He is working tirelessly with hospital fundraisers to develop the capital base he needs to integrate virtual nurses in high-traffic hospital zones. For most of his colleagues, AI feels like science fiction. Of course that's how they would feel. They are used to working with the hospital's antiquated technology. To get everyone used to the idea of updating and upskilling, he starts with an organization-wide change: patient records. As expected, he gets a lot of pushback from staff about the new electronic health record. Mark ignores the groans and complaints. Change is always challenging. It's human nature to want to fall back on old routines. In Mark's experience, organizational change can only happen when leaders push forward through complaints and resistance. He thinks to himself, "Staff inevitably catch up and adjust. What else can they do?"

In the twenty-first century, North American healthcare organizations and the health professionals who work in them experience never-ending change. Change has brought much welcome progress. Standardization of care pathways and administrative processes have improved efficiency and quality on a number of dimensions. Technological advancements and pharmaceutical discoveries have multiplied the cures and treatments professionals can offer to patients (Schoenwald, Eaton Hoagwood, et al. 2010). High-speed digital technologies have enabled healthcare providers to reach remote and under-resourced areas (Wilson 2018). However, these gains also have generated new problems and exacerbated old ones. An overwhelming body of evidence shows that we have not eradicated health inequities. In fact, quite the opposite. Many patients still lack access to the wealth of healthcare offerings. And not all patients feel heard and cared for when they do enter the healthcare system.

Common approaches to organizational change can themselves exacerbate these problems. Patients report feeling objectified as they are ferried about in standardized sequences of care orchestrated to address symptoms and conditions (Hafferty and Light 1995; Stevens 2016; Timmermans and Almeling 2009). They are touched, probed, and manipulated but often not listened to or seen as people (Agledahl, Gulbrandsen, et al. 2011). Some patients tell us that they suffer at the hands of the caring professions, even if they leave the encounter cured (Haque and Waytz 2012). At the same time, health professionals of all kinds and in growing numbers are experiencing the toll of working long hours with fewer and fewer resources (Wallace, Lemaire, and Ghali 2009). They face non-stop demands to incorporate new techniques, new technologies, and new pharmaceuticals into their practice – all in the service of the patient, which makes it difficult to resist or challenge the need for these innovations. They are expected to provide this service with positivity.

Most solutions proposed to tackle workforce burnout and attrition have focused on the wellness and resilience of healthcare providers. Such solutions are mostly ineffective, however, because they do not address the underlying conditions of burnout. Instead, they are experienced as an additional burden and stress by healthcare providers because they call for "self-care." It is becoming evident that effective solutions to burnout require organizational reform (Shanafelt and Noseworthy 2017). Organizations have been called upon to harness the potential of new technologies, establish supportive cultures, streamline operations, and attract compassionate executive leaders (Shanafelt and Noseworthy 2017).

In this chapter, we explore how organizations and their leaders can support compassionate care by attending to technology, structure, culture, and process. We argue that healthcare professionals cannot be compassionate if the organizations they work for are not compassionate to them. We define healthcare organizations as places and spaces where healthcare delivery happens in a systematic and organized way (e.g., hospitals, clinics, hospices, and long-term care homes). When we refer to healthcare personnel, people, or employees, we include healthcare providers, administrative staff, faculty, students, scientists, and other individuals who are directly or indirectly involved in the delivery of care to patients and their families.

Organizations must first confront the challenge of determining *what* exactly is worth reforming. We have learned through empirical research that *compassion* means many things within healthcare discourses: it is variously understood as an intrinsic identity, a learned identity, a finite resource, a performed action, a value, and an obligation (Stergiopoulos, Ellaway, et al. 2019). In practical terms, such multiple meanings can be difficult to work with. Each one implies distinct values and suggests different foci for change efforts. For example, where compassion is understood as something innate to an individual, organizations might naturally focus on hiring procedures to attract compassionate individuals, and collectively they, in turn, will establish a culture of compassion across the organization. Where compassion is understood as a performed action that involves the coordination of different individuals, technologies, policies, and processes across contexts, organizations might focus on establishing better work conditions that encourage and enable healthcare providers to feel and act in caring and compassionate ways across contexts. Such an approach would make caring and compassion part of the broader organizational values and culture for running an institution.

Such diverse courses of action can introduce tensions and confusion; however, they also offer multiple avenues for effecting change. The different interpretations of caring and compassion that permeate healthcare spaces can provide an entry point for defining multi-level reform agendas (Stergiopoulos, Ellaway, et al. 2019). For this reason, the AMS Phoenix Program has engaged in articulating a set of principles that can be used as a compass to guide organizations that want to support caring and compassion. Members of the AMS Phoenix Project senior management committee distilled the findings of the recent empirical work mentioned above (Stergiopoulos, Ellaway, et al. 2019) into a set of principles for reform that incorporated diverse conceptualizations of caring and compassion. In turn, the principles were presented for feedback to the broader AMS community at an annual conference. Healthcare leaders who were not familiar with the AMS vision were also consulted. Feedback from all of the above consultations was synthesized into the full set of principles that appear in table 7.1.

Our goal in this chapter is to elaborate on these guiding principles with explicit focus on the associated programs of action available to organizations that want to support caring and compassion. Our discussion is organized under eight important characteristics of compassionate healthcare organizations and anchored by a series of case examples. Each of the examples illustrates the need for compassionate organizations and suggests how multiple principles and actions converge in practice.

COMPASSIONATE ORGANIZATIONS ACT UPON EXPLICIT COMMITMENTS

Organizations that strive to instill a culture of compassion appreciate that mission statements should be purposeful and deliberate commitments to a way of being, seeing, and acting. It is not the language but the *logic* of caring and compassion that needs to be incorporated into all levels of organizational planning (Dutton, Lilius, and Kanov 2007; Dutton, Worline, et al. 2006). That is a much more effortful task than simply adding a line or two to a mission statement. For example, it entails exploring patient needs regularly and keeping track of how changing demographics might require alterations to who is hired and

Table 7.1
Principles for compassionate healthcare organizations

Priorities	Actions
Person-centred, holistic, and compassionate care	• Engages front-line providers in the development and implementation of caring practices • Facilitates the voices of patients and their families as integral partners in shaping healthcare provider education and practice • Considers the complete person, physically, psychologically, socially, and spiritually, in the administration of the organization and the compassionate management and prevention of illness and disease • Fulfills responsibilities to truth and reconciliation
Compassionate leadership	• Expects leaders to apply compassion in the administration and management of healthcare people • Assesses regularly the compassionate performance of leaders and makes changes to leadership as appropriate • Engages in collaborative decision-making • Promotes flexibility in work arrangements • Supports work and life integration • Validates teamwork in the delivery of care
Safe and health-promoting environments	• Commits to creating and safeguarding safe and respectful workplace environments that support the well-being of all • Offers transparent and accessible frameworks for all to identify, report, and access support for harassment or abuse • Nurtures a culture of safety where it is possible to raise concerns without feeling threatened • Ensures that physical environments are accessible and navigable for people of all abilities, including those who use mobility aides or service animals
Well-being and self-care	• Actively validates and supports all within the organization to consider their own well-being in addition to taking care of patients and families • Develops, evaluates, and continuously improves accessible institutional initiatives for well-being in the workplace (e.g., creating trust and transparency, including healthy and accessible food options, providing quiet spaces, dedicated seminars and training on well-being and self-care)
Caring practices	• Creates structures and conditions to support the delivery of compassionate care by instilling values of collaboration, teamwork, agency, autonomy, and social responsibility across the healthcare organization • Seeks out and applies multiple perspectives on how to deliver compassionate care that meet the needs of diverse patients and their families
Health equity and diversity	• Commits resources and expertise to identify and address health inequities • Remains vigilant about identifying and eradicating discriminatory conduct across the organization predicated on gender, class, race, ability, sexual orientation, and privilege

Priorities	Actions
Health equity and diversity	• Develops skills related to critique and reflexivity in delivery and education • Ensures diverse perspectives are respected and encouraged and facilitates conflict resolution
Organizational culture of compassion	• Incorporates a commitment to caring and compassion in its mission statement • Inspires and nurtures a culture of caring and compassion for all • Includes a recognized commitment to caring and compassion in all recruitment and evaluation practices • Is sensitive to, and works to eliminate, any possible misalignments between organizational policies, priorities, and protocols and the compassionate mission of the organization • Generates evidence of commitment to caring and compassion
Patient engagement	• Recognizes patients and families as foundational to a vision of a compassionate organization and healthcare system • Creates opportunities for respectful and safe engagement of patients and families in health professional care and education • Reflects on and appropriately incorporates feedback from patients and families to improve healthcare delivery and quality
Transparency and accountability to person-centred, holistic, and compassionate care	• Meaningfully incorporates patients' goals and patient-family satisfaction values in physical, mental, emotional, and spiritual domains of well-being • Strives to achieve measurable improvements in the delivery of holistic and compassionate care through healthcare outcomes

reforms in how organizations approach care. It also requires developing spaces for safe and deliberate reflection on the experiences of delivering care, along with capacity to act on mistakes made and lessons learned (de Zulueta 2013; Kahn, Maurer, et al. 2014). These are moments for breaking out of routines and standardized approaches to consider which logic of compassion might apply in a given situation (Martimianakis and Hafferty 2016). The core message is that simply adopting a convincing definition of caring and compassion will not automatically translate into practices that show responsiveness to the needs of all people.

Compassionate organizations must strive to recognize the goals and values of patients and families in physical, mental, emotional, and spiritual domains of well-being at every encounter. This requires judging quality by establishing evaluation practices that capture process dimensions along with health outcomes. They must also endeavour to eliminate discrimination across the organization and show intolerance to working conditions that challenge the capacity of healthcare personnel to make healthy and balanced life choices. Most of all, compassionate organizations should measure success not only in how many patients they have cared for but also in terms of how well cared for patients have felt in their hands. Compassion in healthcare can generate an ongoing struggle of managing and negotiating different meanings and values of what constitutes good health.

"I can't keep up with this pace. Maybe it's time to retire"

Nurse practitioner Stefania has just returned to her unit for work after a short medical leave. Her colleagues are excited to see her back. Everyone had been so supportive while she was away, sending her notes and keeping her abreast of happenings on the ward. They really pulled through when she needed their advice about how to manage cancer treatment. That's all behind her now. She is really happy to be back.

Stefania starts her day as she typically did before she went on leave, only to find that many things have changed. Her hospital launched a new electronic health record platform a couple of months ago. Stefania knew this was coming but missed the pilot phases. She received the mandatory training before she started back to work, but she quickly realizes the training was not enough. Everyone else has had the opportunity to adjust to the new system, and many new routines have been established on the unit. Stefania feels ineffective and compromised in her work. There is so much to learn! Her brain still feels a bit fuzzy from the cancer treatment. She finds she has to double check everything.

Patients and colleagues start showing their irritation as delays pile up. She catches herself losing her patience with one particularly vocal patient who is complaining about how long it took her to complete a task. The most disheartening thing is that the electronic health record was supposed to make things easier and improve patient care. Instead, it has curtailed much of her independence. She needs the attending physician to authorize many tasks that before were left to her to manage. She wonders if coming back was the right decision. Her stress levels are up and she is worried about being able to keep pace. Her family is urging her to take care of herself. She is exhausted. She had forgotten the toll of a regular shift on her body.

A few weeks later, Stefania is on night shift and she is still struggling. She is finding it very difficult to catch up to her colleagues. Her work relationships have started to suffer. She no longer feels comfortable asking for help. Everyone is just so busy, she feels guilty interrupting them to ask questions. Her manager comes by to hand her a flyer about an upcoming workshop that she strongly recommends Stefania attend. The title of the talk is "Improving collegiality through self-care." Stefania wonders if her manager is trying to tell her something. She recalls a few times over the past week when her irritability got the better of her. She suddenly feels drained. She thinks to herself, "I can't keep up with this pace. Maybe it's time to retire."

COMPASSIONATE ORGANIZATIONS SUPPORT SYSTEMIC AND INDIVIDUAL SOLUTIONS TO BURNOUT

Caring work is emotionally, mentally, and physically effortful. Endeavours to transform the organization must account not only for the financial cost but also the toll on personnel and patients. Incorporating innovative solutions requires the careful introduction of new technologies, pharmaceuticals, and management solutions. Implementation of innovations such as new tools and new medicine and changes to organizational infrastructure, policies and processes require continual learning. Staff cannot effectively adapt to change if they have to compromise on the time they need to rest and recharge. The greatest irony is that the more healthcare providers commit and engage with their work, the greater the risk they will burn out, lose their capacity to empathize with the suffering of their patients, and sever the very relationships that give meaning to the terms *compassion* and *caring*. How do we prevent and address this occupational epidemic? Organizations need to care for healthcare providers so that they can optimally care for their patients. The most fundamental shift should be to stop treating the symptoms of burnout solely at the level of individual employees.

All across North America we have wellness movements that target individual occupational health issues. Yoga classes and other approaches to stress relief are currently appearing across healthcare organizations. Such initiatives do show goodwill when they are organized to thank and support employees. However, they can also compound the problem when organizations deploy solutions that treat symptoms without addressing the underlying conditions that lead to occupational burnout. Organizations must avoid inadvertently downloading the responsibility for reform to individuals when the cause of their stress is beyond their control to fix. This is particularly salient in periods of organizational change. Technologies cannot fully address resourcing shortfalls. New technologies afford efficiencies only when organizations have ensured there is appropriate space and time for their introduction.

While healthcare providers are encouraged to "take care of themselves," organizations should commit resources to facilitate this. At a minimum, healthcare employees should have access to information on how to secure counselling for mental health and addictions. Staff benefit packages should include fitness and other health benefits that support preventative healthcare. Organizations should also strive to minimize preventable stressors and establish transformative health systems that are resilient to change. Within such systems, employees can bounce back from adversity, knowing they are not returning to the same situation they were burning out from.

As various chapters in this book have catalogued, the erosion of empathy is a complex phenomenon produced by a combination of personal, organizational, and societal factors. Organizations must therefore take stock of practices that create moral and ethical challenges for employees. For example, organizations should not encourage efficiency at the expense of regular mental and physical breaks for healthcare providers (Lemaire, Wallace, et al. 2011). Healthcare employees and trainees report that in many contexts, taking a bathroom break, stopping to eat lunch, or taking the time to learn a new skill is perceived as slacking when a clinic is busy and patients are waiting. Scheduling meetings over typical breakfast, lunch, or dinner times and not catering meals because of cutbacks puts the onus on employees to find time in an always busy day to meet basic health and nutritional needs.

Organizations should not tolerate a culture where altruism and self-sacrifice are so valued that it becomes normal practice for employees to work when they are sick, miss major family events, not take holidays, skip regular health check-ups, and routinely work overtime to keep up with expectations. Rather, they should actively validate and support everyone within the organization to consider their own well-being in addition to taking care of patients and families. This entails building an organizational culture of trust and transparency, where there is no fear of reprisal, and where it is acceptable to acknowledge one's fatigue or hunger, or the need for a break or extra time to learn a new technology, or the need to leave early to attend a child's recital or tend an ailing parent.

COMPASSIONATE ORGANIZATIONS
PRIORITIZE CARE ABOVE EFFICIENCY

Contemporary models of care have created many efficiencies. In the process, they have sometimes compromised the relational practices that allow patients to feel cared for as unique individuals. Healthcare employees, burdened with meeting time quotas that are designed to save the system money and reduce wait times for patients, often feel they must choose between slowing down and seeing the patient as a person or "efficiently" treating the condition and moving on to the next complaint. A commitment to holistic care requires reducing wait times without compromising the time spent with each individual patient. What is productive for the system is not always efficient for the patient.

While compassionate organizations spend time truly recognizing and addressing patients' unique needs, many expressions of compassion don't require a lot of time. Involving families in patient care can establish relationships that not only benefit providers and patients but also prove efficient in the long run, even when they initially require more time than allotted for a single patient. When patients are treated supportively and holistically, their care is more likely to be effective. Patients are less likely to re-enter the acute care system as they develop positive behaviours, including adherence to management plans and returning for routine follow-up appointments. It is important for organizations to reframe discussions of efficiency so that quality is not seen simply as a measure of how many minutes one spends with a single patient but rather as health outcomes in the broadest sense.

Organizations truly committed to offering compassionate care will address technological, systemic, structural, and cultural conditions that alienate healthcare providers from their work. This requires a type of collective noticing for organization members to keep track of organizational routines that impede providers from expressing compassion when delivering care (Kanov, Maitlis, et al. 2004; Martimianakis and Hafferty 2016). The most fundamental shift would be to develop models of care that encourage healthcare providers to engage with patients and peers as people, even as they go about treating their symptoms and illnesses (Wright and Katz 2018). Allowing for moments of high emotion with patients and time for peer-to-peer support and reflection in difficult cases will go a long way toward both acknowledging the mental and emotional toil of care and helping healthcare providers to foster a culture of resilience.

To be effective, such opportunities must be explicit and protected. The hidden curriculum literature has documented decades of instances where the value-based teaching of the formal curriculum is unravelled in the day-to-day realities of pressured care delivery. The misalignment of our teaching with the realities of work creates identity dissonance for healthcare providers. Either our values are misplaced or we need to reorganize care such that providers can embody those values in practice (Reay and Hinings 2009).

COMPASSIONATE ORGANIZATIONS
HIRE COMPASSIONATE LEADERS

Leading compassionately is an essential component of running a compassionate organization. Compassionate organizations should recruit compassionate leaders both to model how we expect patients to be treated and to apply compassion in the administration and management of healthcare providers (Hymel, Loeppke et al. 2011; Jones, Winch, et al. 2016). Compassionate leaders appreciate the challenges of balancing multiple expectations, often expectations that are fundamentally in tension. They demonstrate how compassionate acts help fulfill the core mission of a healthcare organization (Kanov, Maitlis, et al. 2004). They engage personnel regularly in decision-making and promote flexible work arrangements that support work and life integration. They promote wellness strategies that include eliminating unrealistic work expectations.

Compassionate leaders are also reflective about the power and privilege that accompany their positions. Acknowledging their own privilege allows leaders to appreciate the challenges of employees who suffer discriminatory organizational practices or attempt to advocate for themselves within a large organization. Compassionate leaders continually review how technologies, structures, and processes support or hinder healthcare personnel in the delivery of care (de Zulueta 2013; Kanov, Maitlis, et al. 2004). They use their positions of power to advocate for others. At the same time, they also hold others accountable to the vision and mission of the organization as they, too, submit to the same expectations. They measure their success with indicators that consider the experiences of healthcare employees and that give equal importance to reducing burnout as they do to reducing wait times for patients (Dzau, Kirch, and Nasca 2018). Compassionate leaders promote the conditions that support the delivery of compassionate care by instilling values of collaboration, teamwork, agency, autonomy, and social responsibility across the organization. They foster positive relationships and a compassionate organizational culture.

COMPASSIONATE ORGANIZATIONS CARE FOR PATIENTS IN DIVERSE WAYS

Allowing patients to have agency and voice, to the extent that they feel comfortable, is a basic premise for good patient care in the twenty-first century. However, it is also very difficult to achieve in a system that is not structured to support the conditions for good team practice, let alone incorporate the patient as a member of the team. This creates frustration for both patients and their healthcare providers.

Part of the mechanism that leads to the objectification of patients is the unidirectional gaze of providers. The all-knowing healthcare team draws on their collective expertise to "make sense" of the patient's condition. However, this one-sided conversation can leave patients feeling uncared for, even if they are cured when they leave settings. Compassionate organizations strive to value the perspectives of all providers and also welcome patients themselves as part of the treatment team. Commitment to authentic person-centred care entails amplifying the voices of patients and their families as integral partners in shaping healthcare provider education and practice.

However, individual healthcare providers should not, and cannot, be all things to all people. Rather, healthcare providers should be equipped with the time, space, and tools necessary to ensure that each patient they encounter during the course of their day is invited to help them understand how they would like to be cared for. Technological advancements, mass education, and the preventative medicine movement have given access to health expertise in ways previously unavailable to patients. Such availability of information means that patients often come to healthcare providers with opinions about their care that include preferred treatment plans in addition to culturally specific preferences related to their care. Compassionate organizations create the conditions for involving patients in their care.

Toward this end, organizations across North America have embarked on various patient engagement strategies. There has been a growing movement to "train" patients to act as partners with healthcare organizations. While such movements go a long way to demonstrate organizations' respect for the voice of the patient, Rowland and Johannesen in chapter 2 also make visible the many ways the patient engagement movement can have unintended consequences. For one, patient needs are infinitely variable and patient engagement strategies invite only a handful of patients to represent all patients. In the process of formalizing patient engagement, we run the risk of stifling diversity. Organizations must thus strive to make every patient encounter an opportunity for engaging the individual patient in defining what will constitute "good care" for them.

COMPASSIONATE ORGANIZATIONS INVOLVE PATIENTS AND PROVIDERS IN ORGANIZATIONAL TRANSFORMATION

Transforming healthcare cannot only be a top-down process. Recognizing the agency of all healthcare providers is important for achieving change that is meaningful for everyone in the organization, especially patients. Involving healthcare providers in iterative cycles of priority-setting and implementation serves to knit mission and vision with outcome. Healthcare organizations that create space for employees to participate in the design of change strategies both reinforce and capitalize on the ethos of care that we train healthcare providers to strive for. If we want healthcare providers to respectfully and authentically integrate the voices of patients when devising plans for taking care of their illness, then the same respect should be afforded to them. Point-of-care healthcare workers have an intimate knowledge of day-to-day practices, a form of expertise that is difficult to reproduce around tables of senior executive leadership and corporate boards.

New models of leadership are required if patients are to be engaged in their care and providers are invited to help transform the organization. In addition, as Tassone and colleagues argue in chapter 6, compassionate leadership is not limited to those in positions of authority. Within a compassionate organization, anyone may be empowered to lead. Thus, providers should be encouraged to invite and act upon feedback from patients and families about how to improve health delivery and quality through collaborative decision-making. For this to happen, collaborative leadership must validate a form of teamwork that also involves the patient in thinking about their care. Most importantly, it means the emphasis is not only on improving communication but also on creating the culture and structures to support productive interactions. By situating the interactions between healthcare providers and patients – and among providers themselves – in a broader system of operations, the organization can move beyond targeting individual behaviours. In doing so, it can also work on reforming the technologies, structures, and processes that interfere with the relationship-building necessary for achieving the best version of care for each individual patient and their family. This encompasses such processes as allowing time for new learning, reframing the focus on efficiency to include reducing health inequities and issues of access, selecting technologies constructed to support compassionate care, and making holistic patient- and family-centred care a marker of quality.

"I don't get to park my Parkinson's at home when I have surgery"

Mohammad sat in the surgeon's office awkwardly supporting his left arm. He needed surgery to repair a bad break. His legs started shaking, the tremors a common feature of living with Parkinson's. His case was handled by an expert surgeon who reassured him that his chronic condition would not affect the surgery. Mohammad was not reassured. The slightest change in his routine or diet always affected his symptoms. So he made sure to tell everyone he met during pre-op prep about his condition. He even handed them instructions that his neurologist had given him for post-op management of his meds. People were polite but did not seem to give much attention to his worries. "We repair this type of break regularly," he heard over and over again.

When Mohammad woke up in the recovery room the cramps and stiffness attacking all parts of his body were worse than the pain from the surgery. Just as he had feared, the Parkinson's drugs were not working as they were supposed to. His wife started to massage the stiffness from the muscles and helped him walk around. Every time they stopped the massage and walking, the cramps and pain would return. When the lights started to signal the end of visiting hours, and the nurses began to usher family members out of the recovery room, Mohammad's wife refused to leave, attracting the head nurse's attention.

The head nurse looked at the patient, supported by his wife, and it seemed that for the first time she really saw him for the person he was – middle-aged, tired, uncomfortable, and vulnerable. Mohammad grimaced as the spasms hit again, his movements awkward as he reached out to his wife to steady himself. The nurse realized she did not have a baseline to appreciate what was normal for this patient. And the reality was, if the patient needed constant massage and support to walk around, there were not enough nurses on duty to be able to provide that kind of individualized care. The nurse broke the rules and allowed the patient's wife to stay. It was a long, sleepless night for all of them. Mohammad was miserable, sore, and exhausted. His wife was equally drained. But the morning finally arrived. The surgical fellow cheerfully walked over to the bed to review the chart, check the wound, and discharge the patient.

"Hello," he said. "How is the arm doing?" Mohammad sighed, turned his head away from the fellow, and thought to himself, "What do I have to do to make them see that I don't get to park my Parkinson's at home when I have surgery!"

The doctor's inquiry about the "the arm" tells a vital story. With no conscious intent to do so, the doctor has effectively ignored the patient. The person, for whom "the arm" is the least of his concerns, remains unseen, unheard, uncared for, and dismissed. At best, he is an inconvenience while his arm stands as a tribute to the skill of the surgical team. In the above example, everyone is working to mend the patient's arm to the best of their capacity. How do they know they are doing a good job? They follow protocol and apply the best evidence at hand for how to repair the arm safely and efficiently. The arm is indeed fixed and the patient heals well.

When someone reviews this case in the future, all they will likely see is one more successful surgery. Nowhere will the chart reflect that the patient was miserable in the hospital. The patient felt unsafe. The patient felt unheard. The patient felt vulnerable and sometimes uncared for. Nowhere in the chart will it say that it was the spouse who supported the patient overnight, that the nurse broke protocol to allow this (perhaps the one act of compassion in the story). Nowhere will it be noted that in the end the nurse spent time learning from the spouse how to care for someone with Parkinson's post-operatively, in case staff encounter another case like this in the future. These important messages and indicators of quality are not officially appreciated.

The "system" and its players are pleased with a great and efficient outcome, but the patient and her husband leave the system traumatized and hurt, mistrustful, and hoping that future encounters with the healthcare system can be avoided. These unintended outcomes are as real as the outcome related to the fracture that was, indeed, fixed with skill and efficiency. These unintended outcomes will influence future health-seeking behaviour in ways that serve no one – not the patient and not the healthcare system.

INCLUSION AND EQUITY REQUIRE
MORE THAN POSTERS AND SLOGANS

Delivery of care begins and ends outside the clinic. If we continue to aim at fixing what is broken only at the point of care, we will continue to frustrate both healthcare providers and patients. Our societies are not perfect, and we should not organize healthcare delivery with the false sense that our imperfect society stays outside the clinic when patients arrive to receive care.

"Inclusion requires more than slogans and pretty pictures"

Shawna is a first-year internal medicine resident working on the medicine wards in an academic hospital. For the last two days, every time Shawna has seen her patient in room 311, she has left the room on the verge of tears. She feels humiliated by comments from the patient, who has asked her repeatedly whether she is qualified to handle his care. Every time she enters the room, he does not greet her or make eye contact, and asks when the real doctor will see him. Shawna was one of only two black women in her entire medical school class. She is recognized by her colleagues and supervisors as a highly skilled and compassionate clinician. As a resident, she is responsible for rounding on her patients on the ward, and then presenting their cases to the rest of the medical team to discuss their management plan. Her team consists of two medical students, a senior resident, a fellow, and an attending physician. She feels her team is supportive; however, the volume of work is overwhelming for all of them, and she feels guilty bringing up her concerns when they are all so overloaded.

The next day, the whole team rounds together on their entire list of patients. As they all enter room 311, the patient sees Shawna, but then speaks directly to the attending physician. "Ah, finally – a real doctor.

Doctor, can you please make sure that I don't have to see this girl again; I don't believe she knows how to take care of me. I'd like to see a Caucasian doctor." Shawna feels her team's eyes on her as she looks down quietly. The room is silent as the attending hesitates, trying to weigh what to say next. She does not like seeing Shawna's embarrassment, but she also feels it's important to honour the patient's wishes. Shawna struggles to keep her composure. She glimpses a poster in the hallway celebrating racial diversity: "Believing in equality makes us stronger." She thinks to herself, "Inclusion requires more than slogans and pretty pictures."

Discrimination has been proven to have significant health effects on all people, including healthcare workers and trainees (Cook, Liutkus, et al. 1996; McConnell and Eva 2012; Scambler 2009; Williams, Neighbors, and Jackson 2003). The attending in the above case is caught trying to negotiate between two competing imperatives: honouring the wishes of a patient and advocating for a colleague. A fundamental responsibility for all healthcare organizations should be to foster a safe, health-promoting work environment that values diversity and equity (Scambler 2009). All healthcare employees should feel respected and safe when they come to work. Respect extends to feeling an integral part of the organization regardless of one's sex, gender, class, race, ability, religious affiliation, or other markers of visible or invisible difference (Pattani, Ginsburg, et al. 2018; Shanafelt and Noseworthy 2017). This requires ensuring additional supports for providers and patients who belong to groups designated as vulnerable. In Shawna's case, her colleagues fell into patterns of historical racism when they remained silent in the face of the patient's demand to see a "real doctor," meaning in this case a white doctor. There is no room for racist and other discriminatory behaviours in patient-centred care. Organizations need to provide clarity about such boundaries in their mandates if compassion and caring are to extend to all.

All employees should be able to raise concerns without fear of reprisal (Scambler 2009). Organizations should offer transparent and accessible frameworks for all to report and access support for harassment and abuse at the hands of peers, managers, families, or patients. Organizational language that emphasizes equality instead of equity and a culture that emphasizes sameness over difference often make advocating for these additional supports challenging, particularly by the people who suffer the consequences of discrimination.

The diverse cultural milieu of North American healthcare contexts makes representation an important marker of quality for healthcare organizations. It requires concerted effort to rectify years of health inequities by ensuring that all members of society have equitable access to culturally sensitive healthcare. Organizations must thus work to ensure that all patients see themselves represented in the teams of healthcare providers to whom they entrust their care. A health-promoting, caring, and compassionate organization of the twenty-first century will commit resources and energy to recruit, hire, and most importantly support members of underprivileged groups (Kanov, Maitlis, et al. 2004; Smith 2012). It will also remain vigilant to identify and eradicate discriminatory conduct across an organization premised on gender, class, race, ability, sexual orientation, and privilege.

A healthcare system that trains and hires people of all races, cultures, religions, genders, and abilities sends an important message to all of society about who is valued and who can have voice in shaping what healthcare looks like (Sarason 1977). This is particularly true for marginalized members of society such as Indigenous peoples, who have suffered neglect, violence, and mistreatment at the hands of colonizers and the brand of medicine they bring with them. In Canada for example, this would also include a formal commitment to the Truth and Reconciliation effort to redress the health inequities that plague Indigenous peoples by supporting the training and employment of Indigenous physicians and by integrating Indigenous health perspectives in the operation of hospitals.

In addition to addressing racial, gender, and historical inequities, strategies for promoting accessibility need to be multi-pronged to integrate the physical, psychological, and social needs of people. Accessible workspaces are fundamental for patients, families, and healthcare employees who use mobility aides or service animals. Ensuring such accessibility in both structural and cultural conditions of work will ensure that all employees are able to work under conditions that allow them to apply their full capabilities to the care of patients.

What we are suggesting is a type of reflexivity at the level of organizations, which appreciates that work stress is not only about tasks but also about the social and physical conditions in which these tasks are to be completed. Organizational leaders who want to promote a compassionate culture must take stock of their own assumptions about what constitutes quality, fairness, and due process in cases where exclusion and discrimination are involved. They should work to encourage evaluation of day-to-day routines that may inadvertently disadvantage some groups of employees over others.

For example, interprofessional dynamics are challenged by long-standing and gendered histories of professional hierarchy that determine who is most influential, which in turn impact workplace privilege and reward mechanisms. A legacy of this gendered tradition is seen in current earning patterns across North American healthcare institutions. Female health professionals regularly earn less than their male counterparts (Rimmer 2014). As well, tasks completed by women are often considered less important than tasks typically associated with men. Fewer women make it to senior management positions in healthcare organizations because they lack the exposure and opportunities to build the resumés required to compete for positions at that level (Byerley 2018). Similar discrepancies in the career trajectories of employees belonging to visible minorities are well documented. Acknowledging the existence of these inequities is only the starting point for institutional reform (Smith 2012). Organizations must make themselves accountable to the public and their employees for regular scrutiny on such forms of discrimination. When they do, they also open up the space for the pre-emptive identification of organizational practices that add undue stress to the lives of employees.

CONCLUSION

In this chapter, we have argued that compassionate, caring organizations must devote concerted time and resources to building meaningful relationships between patients and providers, among providers themselves, and between sectors of the health system, which patients must often navigate on their own. Patients and providers need to be involved as partners in designing compassionate systems for this reason – because the outcomes and challenges of compassionate care are often not readily measurable or predictable.

We have also argued that healthcare providers must make their own health a priority and advocate for themselves as passionately as they advocate for their patients. True compassion and care do not always take more time. Rather, compassion can be found in brief moments – moments in which there is a caring touch, a kind word, a gentle smile, laughter, a genuine thank you, I'm sorry, or I appreciate you. While these things don't always take time, they do require a concerted organizational commitment to instill compassion as a value that is woven into the mission and the practices of organizations. Such moments highlight the value of listening, responding, validating, and acknowledging. They recognize that healthcare, when all is said and done, is a profoundly human enterprise. It is a place where certainty and uncertainty, explicitness and implicitness, abundance and scarcity, standardization and individualization all co-exist. These contrasts are always in tension, rarely perfectly balanced, always moving in the spaces between. Indeed, these are the paradoxes that make healthcare a rewarding profession, where reflexivity balances the standardization clinical work.

In our embracing of the technological advances that are, and will continue to be, essential to a modern health delivery system, the loss of compassion is neither necessary nor inevitable. Compassion can and, we argue should, be embraced and should permeate the culture and ethos of the organization in physical and virtual spaces, institutionally and interpersonally. This also requires us to tolerate complexity and paradox. It involves acknowledging that technology, science, and standardization have crucial roles to play, not exclusively or in isolation but rather in tandem with a visible culture of caring and compassion. For organizations that serve patients, make new discoveries, train new professionals, and employ existing ones, embracing compassion is more necessary than ever.

We have offered various strategies for reform that approach the complexity of caring compassionately for diverse people with diverse needs. With the advent of new technologies and scientific discoveries, we will continue to improve our capacity to cure and treat illnesses. Compassionate organizations will adopt this new learning and will use routines, standards of care, and efficiencies to achieve safe and positive clinical outcomes for patients, but they will not make this their mission. Instead, they will treat these operational practices as a stepping stone to achieving their true mission of providing compassionate, person-centred care for all patients and their families.

Shaping the Future of Compassionate Care

Brian D. Hodges, Gail Paech, and Jocelyn Bennett

For over eighty years, AMS Healthcare has been a catalyst organization, striving to decode the future of healthcare and to help leaders prepare. Today we stand at the start of a new revolution. Having spent nearly a decade funding research, innovation, and education in compassionate care, we have come to recognize that emerging technologies present a compelling and urgent imperative to reconsider what healthcare is and what it could become.

The authors in this book articulate a compassionate imperative for healthcare that can guide our way as we navigate technological change. Their contributions crystalize the diverse perspectives and robust expertise of the AMS Phoenix Program. By investing in fellowships, projects, local meetings, and international conferences, this program has established one of the largest communities and bodies of knowledge focused on compassion in healthcare. Complementing this work is an explosion of writing on compassion by educators, evaluators, and policy experts around the world.

This book is our collective call to action. A call to embrace the significant opportunity that technological advancement provides to enhance healthcare systems, Canadian and global. A call to ensure that compassion remains at the centre of healthcare as the technological revolution unfolds. A call for *you* to act by leading from where you stand, whether in education, research, practice, or policy. There is an urgent need for leaders who can think deeply and critically about emerging technologies, about roles we have not yet imagined, about who future healthcare providers will be and what they will do. If healthcare workers, educators, and patients do not engage in wide and careful discussion about the adoption of technologies, technologies will be adopted without us and may operate at cross purposes to care.

Emerging technologies, including machine learning and AI, robotics, and massive databases held in clouds, are already transforming patient lives and healthcare work. Though healthcare has so far been somewhat less affected than the manufacturing, financial, or transportation sectors, change has indeed begun. In the last few years alone, computers equipped with AI have begun to interpret patterns in X-rays, retinal scans, and dermatology images. Genomes can today be scanned in seconds. Mountains of patient information and test results are mined for prognostication.

And then in early 2020, everything changed. It may be that we look back a few years from now and realize that it was a tiny virus – COVID-19 – that gave the most important push to a digital and virtual healthcare transformation. When, for a time, healthcare professionals, patients, and families faced the harsh reality that they could not see each other in person, a phenomenally rapid adoption of technology took place. During a period when personal contact presented a risk of infection, technology has provided a connection. But the rapid immersion into technological-mediated healthcare has also made visible all the pressing issues raised in this book. Many people did not and cannot access computers; digital tools are unequally available. For some, a virtual connection has been a godsend, even life-saving. For others, it has felt like a poor substitute for much-needed human touch and human presence. And for the first time, as countries and governments desperate to control the spread of a deadly pathogen sought to harness technologies to monitor that virus, we have seen how the attraction of digital surveillance extended also to their citizens.

For the optimists, the arrival of this new technological prowess now represents an unprecedented opportunity to overcome chronic weaknesses in healthcare systems: variability, inefficiency, and biases in care. It is possible that emerging technologies will also bolster the ability of professionals, institutions, and systems to provide more compassionate care. For the cynics, however, we have had a glimpse of technology that conjures fear of assembly line healthcare in which patients are dehumanized and the human touch of professionals is marginalized. Which of these visions will come to pass?

HEALTHCARE MUST NEVER LOSE COMPASSION

The editors and authors of this book share the view that to lose compassion in healthcare would be a tragedy. At the same time, we have rejected as overly simplistic the notion that humans are compassionate and machines are not. R. Susskind and D. Susskind (2015, 251) call this the "empathy objection." Professionals, they write, are quick to argue that only humans can convey the empathy required to help a sick patient, troubled client, or distraught student. Yet these authors suggest that professionals overplay the "empathy card." They point to a litany of research showing that many health professionals and institutions are lacking in empathy and that the health professions have openly struggled with this for decades. They argue for caution in expecting more from machines than we do from humans. They point out that empathy has cognitive as well as affective components; machines may well become adept at detecting objective signs and symptoms and responding in ways that help individuals to feel understood, even if the affective dimension of care still requires a human. They cite research showing that in some cases people actually prefer to disclose sensitive information to a machine. Finally, and perhaps most powerfully, they state that despite the "alleged indispensability of empathy in the delivery of professional work," (R. Susskind and D. Susskind 2015, 253) in many cases only privileged individuals can afford and access highly compassionate care.

The example of caring for people with dementia comes to mind. As AI-enabled robotic systems become available, many will claim that such machines can never provide the empathy of a human. But this begs the question of how much of the healthcare labour force is available to care for patients with dementia. It also fails to consider the steep emotional and financial tolls that often fall upon unpaid care providers. Overtaxed personal support workers, healthcare aids, and family caregivers carry the burden around the clock, and are able to access the empathic care of a doctor or nurse only in very short appointments, if at all. Why would a family not want to use a technology that could provide comfort and support?

The authors have therefore troubled the complex relationship between compassion and technology. As Wiljer, Strudwick, and

Crawford write in chapter 1, some technologies can amplify and extend human compassion, making these technologies "empathic" to some degree in their own right. These authors make it clear that whether a healthcare experience is empathetic depends upon the purpose and choices of the healthcare professional, the perceptions of the patient, and a host of other factors. An ecological perspective is necessary to understand the impact that particular technologies will have. A nurse who turns her back on a patient to enter data into a computer has made a choice different from another who invites a patient to look with her at the screen.

The healthcare service she works for has also made a choice: to purchase desktop computers and create office configurations that force clinicians to turn their backs on patients. Imagine, by contrast, a homecare professional equipped by her healthcare agency with a tablet that enables her to sit side by side with a patient, accessing personalized online information and fostering greater understanding and empathy in the process. Through all of these choices, health professionals, institutions, and agencies reveal to what degree their purpose is compassionate. The development of digital compassion frameworks and strategies are tangible leadership actions that can be taken now.

Maunder, Chaukos, and Lawson in chapter 4 broaden the focus by showing how health professionals themselves and the environments in which they work are inseparable from compassionate care. Burnout is rampant in hospitals and clinics but is seldom framed as a problem of technology and compassion. Any consideration of technology is incomplete if it fails to account for the experiences of those who use it. There are important lessons from the widespread adoption of electronic health records, for example. On the one hand, these now ubiquitous systems have greatly streamlined data capture and analysis. On the other hand, they have had deleterious effects on healthcare providers, increasing administrative burden, fostering isolation, and threatening sense of purpose and control. Maunder, Chaukos, and Lawson show us that the development of strong interpersonal relationships and supportive networks allows health professionals to have sufficient "relational reserves" to thrive in highly stressful work environments. These authors suggest how considering the ratios of demand-to-control and effort-to-reward can prevent burnout within service organizations. This framework can be practically and immediately applied to the design and purchase of technologies.

Throughout this book, there has also been vigorous discussion about what compassion *is*. It is not difficult to understand the importance of empathy and caring at the interpersonal level. Many of us engage easily with the idea of compassion in one-to-one interactions between healthcare professionals and patients, as well as those between professionals themselves. But several authors of this book have challenged that scope of compassion as reductionist. Compassion or the lack thereof, they argue, is also a feature of organizations and of whole societies.

Martimianakis and colleagues in chapter 7 show that institutions are themselves a kind of technology. When we walk into a building, a clinic, a hospital, or a long-term care home, our experience is powerfully shaped in the first few minutes. Is it welcoming or does it convey a sense of foreboding? Does it draw us in comfortably or does it project barriers? The way institutions are constructed sends strong messages to those who enter or inhabit them. These messages are equally potent in the virtual spaces that institutions create, such as websites and patient portals. From their entry lobby to their internet spaces, institutions develop cultures that may convey deep and inclusive caring and compassion or something quite different. Martimianakis and her colleagues invite us to open our eyes to see what is around us and redesign what works against compassionate care.

Institutions are not static; they are shaped and reshaped by their leaders. What an institution conveys to those who interact with it derives in large part from the values of its leaders. Chapter 6 by Tassone and colleagues reminds us that we cannot hope to have compassionate care without compassionate leaders. The best writing about leadership also counters a problematic discourse that dismisses compassionate leadership as a soft skill by drawing attention to evidence that leadership practices influence widely valued outcomes such as mortality, patient satisfaction, and malpractice complaints (de Zulueta 2016). Leadership is about attributes and values, not positions or titles. The time is now to develop ways of being and doing that enable us all to lead with compassion.

Among the many voices in this book, perhaps the most troubling appear in chapter 3 by Paton and colleagues. These authors challenge all-too-easy solutions that might enhance the care only of people who can readily access healthcare systems. They tell us that technologies have unequal application and can aggravate socio-economic, cultural, and gender disparities. Focusing on the experience of "the patient" in the abstract obscures the fact that whole populations, such as homeless, Indigenous, immigrant, are not even considered in some constructions of compassionate care. The decisions made about technology can, and must, include the lens of their effect on the broader social good. As these authors write, "Compassionate care will not be established with technology alone, but if deployed with a focus on equity and equitable distribution ... [it] can be more easily realized" (see page 101). Frameworks for the evaluation, acquisition, and deployment of new technologies must today include this perspective.

It is fitting therefore to finish with consideration of the perspective of patients in the broadest sense of the word. The twenty-first century has witnessed a steady rise of patients and families participating in their own healthcare. While notions such as "patient education" and "patient empowerment" were adequate in the twentieth century, today the conversation has changed. The important question no longer concerns the rules by which professionals should share information with patients. Instead, it concerns who owns the information in the first place. Traditionally, paternalistic health professionals meted out bits of information they thought patients and families should know. Today, patients want to control their own destiny. This entails accessing and controlling their own healthcare data: how it is held, manipulated, studied, aggregated, and shared. As these functions increasingly involve technologies like AI, patients must be involved in system design.

Rowland and Johannesen show in chapter 2 that patient engagement programs are themselves technologies, and are often instrumental and technocratic. Whether such approaches are compassionate is in question. The shape they take in healthcare settings hinges on what individuals and institutions believe suffering is. These authors argue that health professionals too easily identify their compassionate purpose as reducing suffering through treatments and cures. The enormous efforts currently underway to harness data-driven technologies largely have a curative orientation. Yet, patients and families experience many things for which there is no fix; no data, no analysis, no AI will help. In other words, the "taking action" that has underpinned the definition of compassion throughout this book may sometimes consist of doing nothing more than bearing witness to existential suffering. Bearing witness, they remind us, requires human presence and human time.

TIME

That brings us to a last and crucial idea. Eric Topol, author of *Deep Medicine* (2019a), subtitled his book "How Artificial Intelligence Can Make Healthcare Human Again." Though his analysis of the many applications of AI is detailed, Topol's main argument is that AI will enhance humanism by providing the "gift of time." He invited noted medical humanist Dr Abraham Verghese to write the foreword to the book. Verghese provides a strong case for empathy, compassion, and human presence. However, he also makes clear that Topol's argument rests on a big *if*. AI *may* enhance the compassionate care of patients *if* the time found through automation is reinvested in human interaction. Topol expands: "AI is going to profoundly change medicine. That doesn't necessarily mean for the better" (Topol 2019a, 285).

We editors of this book have significant experience in the management of healthcare systems and deeply share this concern. Our own experiences have taught us how difficult it is to protect and reinvest "found" time, even if it is made available, in an overburdened healthcare system. Topol paints a picture in which automation, improved diagnosis, and treatment aided by AI almost certainly will free up time, but he concedes that, "[t]he super-streamlined workflow that lies before us, affecting every aspect of healthcare as we know it today in one way or another, could be used in two very different, opposing ways: to make things much better or far worse. We have to get out in front of it now to be sure this goes in the right direction" (Topol 2019a, 285).

This book is a first step to "getting out in front."

GETTING OUT IN FRONT: EDUCATION REFORM

In the 1980s, AMS Healthcare led one of the largest population-based studies ever conducted to understand what patients expect from their physicians. The project was called "Educating Future Physicians for Ontario," and it produced a framework that, with refinement from the Royal College of Physicians and Surgeons of Canada, would become the "CanMEDs competence framework." Today this framework has been adopted around the world and by myriad health professions. What was the magic of this framework? In articulating what the Canadian public expected of their health professionals – to be adept in communication, collaboration, advocacy, leadership, and scholarship as well as clinical expertise – the framework greatly broadened how educators prepared future health professionals (Frank and Danoff 2007; Frank, Jabbour, and Tugwell 1996; Neufeld, Maudsley, et al. 1993).

As we enter the third decade of the twenty-first century, it is once again time to recalibrate health professional education. Mallette, Rose, and Spadoni in chapter 5 illustrate powerfully the daunting challenge today's educators face in preparing themselves and their students for an uncertain future. Competencies such as metacognition,[1] collaboration with machines, human-machine integration, and the humane uses of technology must urgently be incorporated. Tomorrow's healthcare professionals must be capable of navigating complex, uncertain environments. Given how much is unforeseeable, curious and reflective practitioners, educators, and leaders must be identified and nurtured. Tomorrow's healthcare teams must be trained today. They will include those who work with advanced technologies (like the personal support worker, also known as P S W, who uses smart phone–driven wound analysis and communications devices to provide care at home), as well as the technologies themselves (like the AI-enabled robot) – the newest members of the surgical or rehabilitation team.

All of these advances and applications have profound implications for education. Starting with this book, A M S Healthcare will "get out in front," launching a national dialogue and a call to action to once again reform health professional education. The time is now to adapt admissions, curricula, standards, certification, and lifelong learning to meet the future needs of our societies.

WILL TECHNOLOGY UNLOCK HUMAN COMPASSION?

So we end where we began. Was Bill Gates right to say that technology will unlock human compassion, or rather the Dalai Lama to say that technology will never replace it? The editors and authors of this book go beyond that dated dichotomy. Ursula Franklin (1999, 25), in her foresighted book *The Real World of Technology*, writes: "If we do not wish to visualize people as sources of problems and machines as sources of solutions, then we need to consider machines and devices as cohabitants of this earth." While machines cannot be made human, and humans should not be driven to be machine-like, compassionate healthcare will be sustained only by helping people who provide it to access the most human parts of themselves and to extend their compassionate impulses through human-created and human-governed technologies.

Regardless of the path ahead, human health professionals must redouble efforts to anchor healthcare in compassion: it is a covenant that has served across countless ages. Whether harnessing spirits or giving medicines, whether cutting with blades or calming with talk, whether vaccinating an anxious child or simply holding the hand of a distraught senior, everything health professionals do must be anchored in compassion. During the COVID-19 crisis, people have reacted with horror at the thought of seniors, permitted no visitors, dying alone in institutions. Necessity led to creative uses of digital tools to make connections, streaming digital voices and images. But perhaps the most moving stories of hope and compassion involved nurses and PSWs, present in hospitals, ICUs, and long-term care homes, to hold the hands of people in their final moments. If computers equipped with AI, or robots, or enormous banks of data can help us with these crucial human connections and convey essential human presence, so much the better. But in adopting sparkly new technologies, the compassionate purpose of healthcare must never be lost. While efficiency, quality, safety, accessibility, and a myriad of performance indicators are critical, without compassion, they will not be healthcare.

NOTE

1 According to Lexico.com (2020), metacognition is an awareness and understanding of one's own thought processes.

References

Abelson, Julia, Pierre-Gerlier Forest, John Eyles, Patricia Smith, Elisabeth Martin, and Francois-Pierre Gauvin. 2003. "Deliberations about Deliberative Methods: Issues in the Design and Evaluation of Public Participation Processes." *Social Science & Medicine* 57 (2): 239–51. doi: 10.1016/s0277-9536(02)00343-x.

Adams, Howard. 1975. *Prison of Grass: Canada from a Native Point of View*. Saskatoon: Fifth House Publishers.

Adriaenssens, Jef, Véronique de Gucht, and Stan Maes. 2015. "Determinants and Prevalence of Burnout in Emergency Nurses: A Systematic Review of 25 Years of Research." *Int J Nurs Stud* 52 (2): 649–61. doi: 10.1016/j.ijnurstu.2014.11.004.

Agledahl, Kari Milch, Pål Gulbrandsen, Reidun Førde, and Åge Wifstad. 2011. "Courteous but Not Curious: How Doctors' Politeness Masks Their Existential Neglect. A Qualitative Study of Video-Recorded Patient Consultations." *Journal of Medical Ethics* 37 (11): 650–4. doi: 10.1136/jme.2010.041988.

Agrawal, Ajay, Joshua Gans, and Avi Goldfarb. 2018. *Prediction Machines*. Boston: Harvard Business Review Press.

Ahola, Kirsi, and Jari Hakanen. 2007. "Job Strain, Burnout, and Depressive Symptoms: A Prospective Study among Dentists." *J Affect Disord* 104 (1–3): 103–10. doi: 10.1016/j.jad.2007.03.004.

Aiken, Linda H., Sean P. Clarke, Douglas M. Sloane, Julie Sochalski, and Jeffrey H. Silber. 2002. "Hospital Nurse Staffing and Patient Mortality, Nurse Burnout, and Job Dissatisfaction." *Journal of the American Medical Association* 288 (16): 1987–93. doi: 10.1001/jama.288.16.1987.

Aiken, Linda H., Herbert L. Smith, and Eileen T. Lake. 1994. "Lower
  Medicare Mortality among a Set of Hospitals Known for Good Nursing
  Care." *Med. Care* 32 (8):771–87.
Ali, Sulekha, and Louise Terry. 2017. "Exploring Senior Nurses' Under-
  standing of Compassionate Leadership in the Community." *British
  Journal of Community Nursing* 22 (2):77–87. doi: 10.12968/
  bjcn.2017.22.2.77.
Almendrala, Anna. 2014. "Dalai Lama on Hollywood: It's Bad for
  My Eyes and a Waste of Time." *Huffington Post*, 26 February 2014.
Almerud, Sofia, Richard J. Alapack, Bengt Fridlund, and Margaretha
  Ekebergh. 2008. "Beleaguered by Technology: Care in Technologically
  Intense Environments." *Nursing Philosophy* 9 (1):55–61. doi: 10.1111/
  j.1466-769X.2007.00332.x.
Amoafo, E., N. Hanbali, A. Patel, and Priyanka Singh. 2015. "What
  Are the Significant Factors Associated with Burnout in Doctors?"
  Occup Med (Lond) 65 (2): 117–21. doi: 10.1093/occmed/kqu144.
Andrews, Jason R., Robin Wood, Linda-Gail Bekker, Keren Middelkoop,
  and Rochelle P. Walensky. 2012. "Projecting the Benefits of
  Antiretroviral Therapy for HIV Prevention: The Impact of Population
  Mobility and Linkage to Care." *The Journal of Infectious Diseases*
  206 (4): 543–51.
Arndt, Brian G., John W. Beasley, Michelle D. Watkinson, Jonathan L.
  Temte, Wen-Jan Tuan, Christine A. Sinsky, and Valerie J. Gilchrist. 2017.
  "Tethered to the EHR: Primary Care Physician Workload Assessment
  Using EHR Event Log Data and Time-Motion Observations." *Ann Fam
  Med* 15 (5): 419–26.
Arnold, Elizabeth C., and Kathleen Underman Boggs. 2019. *Interpersonal
  Relationships E-Book: Professional Communication Skills for Nurses.*
  8th ed. St Louis: Elsevier Health Sciences.
Arrigoni, Cristina, Rosaria Alvaro, Ercole Vellone, and Marina Vanzetta.
  2016. "Social Media and Nurse Education: An Integrative Review of
  the Literature." *Journal of Mass Communication & Journalism* 6 (1):
  290–7. doi: 10.4172/2165-7912.1000290.
Arthur, Emily, Amanda Seymour, Michelle Dartnall, Paula Beltgens, Nancy
  Poole, Diane Smylie, Naomi North, Rose Schmidt, Cristine Urquhart,
  and Fran Jasiur. 2013. *Trauma Informed Practice Guide.* Vancouver:
  British Columbia Centre of Excellence for Women's Health.
Associated Medical Services. 2017. *Transformational Trends in Healthcare.*
  Toronto: Associated Medical Services. http://www.ams-inc.on.ca/
  wp-content/uploads/2015/12/Future-Trends-That-are-Transforming-
  Healthcare.pdf.

Atkins, Paul W., and Sharon K. Parker. 2012. "Understanding Individual Compassion in Organizations: The Role of Appraisals and Psychological Flexibility." *Academy of Management Review* 37 (4): 524–46. doi: 10.5465/arar.2010.0490.

Avery, Emily, and Jocalyn Clark. 2016. "Sex-Related Reporting in Randomised Controlled Trials in Medical Journals." *Lancet* 388 (10062): 2839–40. doi: 10.1016/s0140-6736(16)32393-5.

Awa, Wendy L., Martina Plaumann, and Ulla Walter. 2010. "Burnout Prevention: A Review of Intervention Programs." *Patient Educ Couns* 78 (2): 184–90. doi: 10.1016/j.pec.2009.04.008.

Ayalon, Liat 2008. "Subjective Socioeconomic Status as a Predictor of Long-Term Care Staff Burnout and Positive Caregiving Experiences." *Int Psychogeriatr* 20 (3): 521–37. doi: 10.1017/S1041610207006175.

Baker, J.I. 2018. "The Digital-Era Brain." *Time Special Edition, The Science of Memory: The Story of Our Lives*, 21 December 2018, 62–5.

Barnard, Alan. 2016. "Radical Nursing and the Emergence of Technique as Healthcare Technology." *Nursing Philosophy* 17 (1): 8–18. doi: 10.1111/nup.12103.

Bell Let's Talk. 2019. "Growing the Global Conversation and Supporting Canada's Mental Health." https://letstalk.bell.ca/en/results-impact/.

Benjamin, Ruha. 2013. *People's Science: Bodies and Rights on the Stem Cell Frontier*. Stanford: Stanford University Press.

– ed. 2019. *Captivating Technology: Race, Carceral Technoscience, and Liberatory Imagination in Everyday Life*. Durham: Duke University Press.

Benner, Patricia. 1984. *From Novice to Expert, Excellence and Power in Clinical Nursing Practice*. Menlo Park, CA: Addison-Wesley.

Benson, Nicole M., Deanna Chaukos, Heather Vestal, Emma F. Chad-Friedman, John W. Denninger, and Christina P.C. Borba. 2018. "A Qualitative Analysis of Stress and Relaxation Themes Contributing to Burnout in First-Year Psychiatry and Medicine Residents." *Acad Psychiatry* 42 (5): 630–35. doi: 10.1007/s40596-018-0934-2.

Bergerum, Carolina, Johan Thor, Karin Josefsson, and Maria Wolmesjö. 2019. "How Might Patient Involvement in Healthcare Quality Improvement Efforts Work: A Realist Literature Review." *Health Expectations* 22:952–64. doi: 10.1111/hex.12900.

Bernstein, Lenny. 2016. "Has the Stethoscope Had its Day?" *Guardian*, 9 January 2016.

Bertino, Elisa, Latifur R. Khan, Ravi Sandhu, and Bhavani Thuraisingham. 2006. "Secure Knowledge Management: Confidentiality, Trust, and Privacy." *IEEE Transactions on Systems, Man, and Cybernetics-Part A: Systems and Humans* 36 (3): 429–38. doi: 10.1109/tsmca.2006.871796.

Berwick, Donald M. 2009. "What 'Patient-Centered' Should Mean: Confessions of an Extremist." *Health Affairs* 28 (4): w555–w565. doi: 10.1377/hlthaff.28.4.w555.

Bhatia, R. Sacha, and William Falk. 2018. "Modernizing Canada's Healthcare System through the Virtualization of Services." In *C.D. Howe Institute e-Brief 277*.

Biko, Steve. 2015. *I Write What I Like: Selected Writings*. Chicago: University of Chicago Press.

Bloom, David.E., Elizabeth T. Cafiero, Eva Jané-Llopis, Shafika Abrahams-Gessel, Lakshmi R. Bloom, S. Fathima, Andrea B. Feigl, et al. 2011. *The Global Economic Burden of Non-communicable Diseases*. Geneva: World Economic Forum.

Bloom, Paul. 2017. *Against Empathy: The Case for Rational Compassion*. New York: Random House.

Bohm, David. 1996. *On Dialogue*. New York: Routledge.

Booth, Richard G. 2016. "Informatics and Nursing in a Post-Nursing Informatics World: Future Directions for Nurses in an Automated, Artificially Intelligent, Social-Networked Healthcare Environment." *Canadian Journal of Nursing Leadership* 28 (4): 61–9. doi: 10.12927/cjnl.2016.24563.

Bottomley, John, and Mary Tehan. 2006. "They Don't Know What to Say or Do!" East Melbourne: Palliative Care Victoria.

Bourgeois, Annie-Claude C., M. Edmunds, Amnan Awan, Leigh Jonah, Olivia Varsaneux, and Winnie Siu. 2017. "HIV in Canada – Surveillance Report, 2016." *Canada Communicable Disease Report / Releve des maladies transmissibles au Canada* 43 (12): 248–56.

Boyatzis, Richarc, and Annie McKee. 2005. *Resonant Leadership: Renewing Yourself and Connecting with Others through Mindfulness, Hope, and Compassion*. Boston: Harvard Business School Press.

Bracken, Michele I., Jill T. Messing, Jacquelyn C. Campbell, Lareina N. La Flair, and Joan Kub. 2010. "Intimate Partner Violence and Abuse among Female Nurses and Nursing Personnel: Prevalence and Risk Factors." *Issues Ment Health Nurs* 31 (2): 137–48. doi: 10.3109/01612840903470609.

Brewin, Chris R., Bernice Andrews, and John D. Valentine. 2000. "Meta-analysis of Risk Factors for Posttraumatic Stress Disorder in Trauma-Exposed Adults." *J Consult Clin Psychol* 68 (5):748–66. doi: 10.1037/0022-006x.68.5.748.

Bristow, William. 2011. "Enlightenment." In *Stanford Encyclopedia of Philosophy*. https://plato.stanford.edu/archives/sum2011/entries/enlightenment/.

Brown, Eileen. 2017. "Can Computers Detect Emotion and Predict How People Will React?" *ZDNet*, 3 November 2017.

Brown, Loraine P. 2011. "Revisiting Our Roots: Caring in Nursing Curriculum Design." *Nurse Education in Practice* 11 (6): 360–4. doi: 10.1016/j.nepr.2011.03.007.

Bruce, Judith C. 2018. "Nursing in the 21st Century – Challenging Its Values and Roles." *Professional Nursing Today* 22 (1): 44–8.

Bushe, Gervase R. 2012. "Appreciative Inquiry: Theory and Critique." In *The Routledge Companion To Organizational Change*, edited by David Boje, Bernard Burnes, and John Hassard, 87–103. Oxford, UK: Routledge.

Byerley, Julie Story. 2018. "Mentoring in the Era of #MeToo." *JAMA* 319 (12): 1199–1200. doi: 10.1001/jama.2018.2128.

Canada Health Infoway. 2018a. "Faculty Peer Network Program." Accessed February 2018. https://www.infoway-inforoute.ca/en/our-partners/clinicians-and-the-health-care-community/faculty-peer-network-program.

– 2018b. "What Is Digital Health?" Accessed February 2018. https://www.infoway-inforoute.ca/en/what-we-do/digital-health-and-you/what-is-digital-health.

Canada, Parliament, Senate. Standing Senate Committee on Social Affairs Science and Technology. 2017. *Challenge Ahead: Integrating Robotics, Artificial Intelligence and 3D Printing Technologies into Canada's Healthcare System*. Ottawa, Ontario.

Canadas-De la Fuente, Guillermo A., Cristina Vargas, Concepción San Luis, Immaculada Garcia, Gustavo R. Canadas, and Emilia I. De la Fuente. 2015. "Risk Factors and Prevalence of Burnout Syndrome in the Nursing Profession." *Int J Nurs Stud* 52 (1): 240–9. doi: 10.1016/j.ijnurstu.2014.07.001.

Caputo, John D. 1978. *The Mystical Element in Heidegger's Thought.* Athens: Ohio University Press.

– 1988. *Radical Hermeneutics: Repetition, Deconstruction, and the Hermeneutic Project.* Bloomington: Indiana University Press.

– 2018. *Hermeneutics: Facts and Interpretation in the Age of Information.* London: Penguin UK.

Carbado, Devon W., Kimberlé Williams Crenshaw, Vickie M. Mays, and Barbara Tomlinson. 2013. "Intersectionality." *Du Bois Review: Social Science Research on Race* 10 (2): 303–12. doi: 10.1017/S1742058X13000349.

Cassell, Eric. 1982. "The Nature of Suffering and the Goals of Medicine." *New England Journal of Medicine* 306 (11): 639–45.

Catalani, Caricia, William Philbrick, Hamish Fraser, Patricia Mechael, and Dennis M. Israelski. 2013. "mHealth for HIV Treatment & Prevention: A Systematic Review of the Literature." *The Open AIDS Journal* 7:17–41. doi: 10.2174/1874613620130812003.

CBC Radio. 2018. "White Coat, Black Art: Why This Doctor Went Public with Her Story of Burnout." CBC Radio. Accessed 5 December 2018. https://www.cbc.ca/radio/whitecoat/why-this-doctor-went-public-with-her-story-of-burnout-1.4395640.

– 2019. "A Doctor's Quest to Understand Why so Many Physicians Die by Suicide." CBC Radio. Accessed 27 May 2019. https://www.cbc.ca/radio/outintheopen/helplessness-1.5009529/a-doctor-s-quest-to-understand-why-so-many-physicians-die-by-suicide-1.5028162.

Chang, Feng, and Nishi Gupta. 2015. "Progress in Electronic Medical Record Adoption in Canada." *Canadian Family Physician* 61 (12): 1076–84.

Chataway, Joanna, Rebecca Hanlin, and Raphael Kaplinsky. 2014. "Inclusive Innovation: An Architecture for Policy Development." *Innovation and Development* 4 (1): 33–54. doi: 10.1080/2157930X.2013.876800.

Christiansen, Angela, Mary R. O'Brien, Jennifer A. Kirton, Kate Zubairu, and Lucy Bray. 2015. "Delivering Compassionate Care: The Enablers and Barriers." *British Journal of Nursing* 24 (16): 833–7.

Christopoulos, Katerina A., William E. Cunningham, Curt G. Beckwith, Irene Kuo, Carol E. Golin, Kevin Knight, Patrick M. Flynn, Anne C. Spaulding, Lara S. Coffin, and Bridget Kruszka. 2017. "Lessons Learned from the Implementation of Seek, Test, Treat, Retain Interventions Using Mobile Phones and Text Messaging to Improve Engagement in HIV Care for Vulnerable Populations in the United States." *AIDS and Behavior* 21 (11): 3182–93.

Cislak, Aleksandra, Magdalena Formanowicz, and Tamar Saguy. 2018. "Bias Against Research on Gender Bias." *Scientometrics* 115 (1): 189–200. doi: 10.1007/s11192-018-2667-0.

Cohen, Sheldon, and S. Leonard Syme. 1985. *Social Support and Health*. Orlando: Academic Press.

Coiera, Enrico. 2015. *Guide to Health Informatics*. 3rd ed. Boca Raton: CRC Press.

Cole, Marilyn., and Valnere McLean. 2003. "Therapeutic Relationships Re-defined." *Occupational Therapy in Mental Health* 19 (2): 33–56. doi: 10.1300/J004v19n02_03.

Cook, D.J., J.F. Liutkus, C.L. Risdon, L.E. Griffith, G.H. Guyatt, and S.D. Walter. 1996. "Residents' Experiences of Abuse, Discrimination and Sexual Harassment during Residency Training. McMaster University Residency Training Programs." *CMAJ* 154 (11): 1657–65.

Cooperrider, David, and Diana Whitney. 2005. *Appreciative Inquiry: A Positive Revolution in Change.* San Francisco: Berrett-Koehler Publishers.

Coyle, Joanne. 1999. "Exploring the Meaning of 'Dissatisfaction' with Health Care: The Importance of 'Personal Identity Threat.'" *Sociology of Health & Illness* 21 (1): 95–123. doi: 10.1111/1467-9566. t01-1-00144.

Crawford, Allison, Nadiya Sunderji, Eva Serhal, and John Teshima. 2017. "Proposed Competencies for Providing Integrated Care via Telepsychiatry." *Journal of Technology in Behavioral Science* 2 (1): 1–4.

Crawford, Paul. 2011. "NHS Failures in Care for the Elderly Demand Prompt Remedies." Letter to the Editor. *The Times*, 14 October, 35.

Crawford, Paul, Brian Brown, Marit Kvangarsnes, and Paul Gilbert. 2014. "The Design of Compassionate Care." *Journal of Clinical Nursing* 23 (23–24): 3589–99.

Cribb, Alan. 2017. *Healthcare in Transition: Understanding Key Ideas and Tensions in Contemporary Health Policy.* Chicago: University of Chicago Press.

– 2018. "Improvement Science Meets Improvement Scholarship: Reframing Research for Better Healthcare." *Health Care Anal* 26 (2): 109–23. doi: 10.1007/s10728-017-0354-6.

Crowe, Remle P., Julie K. Bower, Rebecca E. Cash, Ashish R. Panchal, Severo A. Rodriguez, and Susan E. Olivo-Marston. 2018. "Association of Burnout with Workforce-Reducing Factors among EMS Professionals." *Prehosp Emerg Care* 22 (2): 229–36. doi: 10.1080/10903127.2017.1356411.

Dall'Ora, Chiara, Peter Griffiths, Jane Ball, Michael Simon, and Linda H. Aiken. 2015. "Association of 12 h Shifts and Nurses' Job Satisfaction, Burnout and Intention to Leave: Findings from a Cross-Sectional Study of 12 European Countries." *BMJ Open* 5 (9): e008331. doi: 10.1136/bmjopen-2015-008331.

Damschroder, Laura J., David C. Aron, Rosalind E. Keith, Susan R. Kirsh, Jeffery A. Alexander, and Julie C. Lowery. 2009. "Fostering Implementation of Health Services Research Findings into Practice: A Consolidated Framework for Advancing Implementation Science." *Implementation Science* 4 (1): 50.

Daugherty, Paul R., and H. James Wilson. 2018. *Human+ Machine: Reimagining Work in the Age of AI.* Brighton, MA: Harvard Business Press.

Day, Suzanne, Robin Mason, Stephanie Lagosky, and Paula A. Rochon.
2016. "Integrating and Evaluating Sex and Gender in Health Research."
Health Research Policy and Systems 14 (1): 75. doi: 10.1186/
s12961-016-0147-7.

De Saint-Exupéry, Antoine. 1950. *The Wisdom of the Sands*. New York:
Harcourt, Brace.

De Sousa Santos, Boaventura. 2008. *Another Knowledge Is Possible:
Beyond Northern Epistemologies*. London: Verso.

De Zulueta, Paquita. 2013. "Compassion in 21st Century Medicine:
Is It Sustainable?" *Clinical Ethics* 8 (4): 119–28. doi: 10.1177/
1477750913502623.

– 2016. "Developing Compassionate Leadership in Health Care:
An Integrative Review." *Journal of Healthcare Leaders* 8:1–10.
doi: 10.2147/JHL.S93724.

Deeks, Steven G., Sharon R. Lewin, and Diane V. Havlir. 2013. "The End
of AIDS: HIV Infection as a Chronic Disease." *Lancet* 382 (9903):
1525–33. doi: 10.1016/S0140-6736(13)61809-7.

Dei, George J. Sefa, and Gurpreet Singh Johal. 2005. *Critical Issues
in Anti-racist Research Methodologies, Counterpoints*. New York:
P. Lang.

Dewa, Carolyn S., Desmond Loong, Sarah Bonato, Nguyen X. Thanh, and
Philip Jacobs. 2014. "How Does Burnout Affect Physician Productivity?
A Systematic Literature Review." *BMC Health Serv Res* 14:325.
doi: 10.1186/1472-6963-14-325.

Dewar, Belinda. 2013. "Cultivating Compassionate Care." *Nursing
Standard (through 2013)* 27 (34): 48.

Dewar, Belinda, Elizabeth Adamson, Stephen Smith, Joyce Surfleet, and
Linda King. 2014. "Clarifying Misconceptions about Compassionate
Care." *Journal of Advanced Nursing* 70 (8): 1738–47.

Dorward, Jienchi, Tonderai Mabuto, Salome Charalambous, Katherine L.
Fielding, and Christopher J. Hoffmann. 2017. "Factors Associated with
Poor Linkage to HIV Care in South Africa: Secondary Analysis of Data
from the Thol'impilo Trial." *JAIDS Journal of Acquired Immune
Deficiency Syndromes* 76 (5): 453–60. doi: 10.1097/
qai.0000000000001550.

Duffy, Farifteh F., Laura J. Fochtmann, Diana E. Clarke, Keila Barber,
Seung Hee Hong, Joel Yager, Eve K. Mościcki, and Robert M. Plovnick.
2016. "Psychiatrists' Comfort Using Computers and Other Electronic
Devices in Clinical Practice." *Psychiatric Quarterly* 87 (3): 571–84.
doi: 10.1007/s11126-015-9410-2.

Durkin, Mark, Russell Gurbutt, and Jerome Carson. 2018. "Qualities, Teaching, and Measurement of Compassion in Nursing: A Systematic Review." *Nurse Education Today* 63:50–8.

Durning, Steven J., Michelle Costanzo, Anthony R. Artino, Jr., Liselotte N. Dyrbye, Thomas. J. Beckman, Lambert Schuwirth, Eric Holmboe, et al. 2013. "Functional Neuroimaging Correlates of Burnout among Internal Medicine Residents and Faculty Members." *Front Psychiatry* 4:131. doi: 10.3389/fpsyt.2013.00131.

Dutton, Jane E., Jacoba Lilius, and J. Kanov. 2007. "The Transformative Potential of Compassion at Work." In *Handbook of Transformative Cooperation: New Designs and Dynamics*, 107–26. Stanford: Stanford University Press.

Dutton, Jane E., K.M. Workman, and A.E. Hardin. 2014. "Compassion at Work." *Annual Review of Organizational Psychology and Organizational Behavior* 1:277–304. doi: 10.1146/annurev-orgpsych-031413-091221.

Dutton, Jane E., Monica C. Worline, Peter J. Frost, and Jacoba Lilius. 2006. "Explaining Compassion Organizing." *Administrative Science Quarterly* 51 (1): 59–96. doi: 10.2189/asqu.51.1.59.

Dyrbye, Liselotte. N., Coliln P. West, Daniel V. Satele, Sonja Boone, Litjen L.J. Tan, Jeff A. Sloan, and Tait D. Shanafelt. 2014. "Burnout among U.S. Medical Students, Residents, and Early Career Physicians Relative to the General U.S. Population." *Acad Med* 89 (3): 443–51. doi: 10.1097/ACM.0000000000000134.

Dzau, Victor J., Darrell G. Kirch, and Thomas J. Nasca. 2018. "To Care Is Human – Collectively Confronting the Clinician-Burnout Crisis." *The New England Journal of Medicine* 378 (4): 312–14. doi: 10.1056/NEJMp1715127.

Eisenstein, Leo 2018. "To Fight Burnout, Organize." *N Engl J Med* 379 (6): 509–11. doi: 10.1056/NEJMp1803771.

Ellaway, Rachel H., Janet Coral, David Topps, and Maureen Topps. 2015. "Exploring Digital Professionalism." *Medical Teacher* 37 (9): 844–9.

Ellis, Jackie, Mark Cobb, Tina O'Connor, Laurie Dunn, Greg Irving, and Mari Lloyd-Williams. 2015. "The Meaning of Suffering in Patients with Advanced Progressive Cancer." *Chronic Illness* 11 (3): 198–209.

Ellsberg, Mary, Henrica A.F.M. Jansen, Lori Heise, Charlotte H. Watts, and Claudia Garcia-Moreno. 2008. "Intimate Partner Violence and Women's Physical and Mental Health in the WHO Multi-country Study on Women's Health and Domestic Violence: An Observational Study." *Lancet* 371 (9619): 1165–72. doi: https://doi.org/10.1016/S0140-6736(08)60522-X.

Elovainio, Marco, Mika Kivimaki, and Jussi Vahtera. 2002. "Organizational Justice: Evidence of a New Psychosocial Predictor of Health." *Am J Public Health* 92 (1): 105–8.

Esteva, Andre, Brett Kuprel, Roberto A. Novoa, Justin Ko, Susan M. Swetter, Helen M. Blau, and Sebastian Thrun. 2017. "Dermatologist-Level Classification of Skin Cancer with Deep Neural Networks." *Nature* 542 (7639): 115.

Eubanks, Virginia. 2018. *Automating Inequality: How High-Tech Tools Profile, Police, and Punish the Poor*. New York: St. Martin's Press.

FDA (Food and Drug Administration). 2019. "Artificial Intelligence and Machine Learning in Software as a Medical Device." Last modified 6 June 2019. https://www.fda.gov/medical-devices/software-medical-device-samd/artificial-intelligence-and-machine-learning-software-medical-device.

Feeley, Derek. 2017. "The Triple Aim or the Quadruple Aim? Four Points to Help Set Your Strategy." Accessed 15 February 2019. http://www.ihi.org/communities/blogs/the-triple-aim-or-the-quadruple-aim-four-points-to-help-set-your-strategy.

Felblinger, Dianne M. 2011. "Incivility and Bullying in the Nursing Workplace." In *Handbook of Stress in the Occupations*, edited by Janice Langan-Fox and Cary L. Cooper, 5–15. Cheltenham, UK: Edward Elgar.

Ferrarese, Alessia, Giadi Pozzi, Felice Borghi, Alessandro Marano, Paola Delbon, Bruno Amato, Michele. Santangelo, et al. 2016. "Malfunctions of Robotic System in Surgery: Role and Responsibility of Surgeon in Legal Point of View." *Open Med (Wars)* 11 (1): 286–91. doi: 10.1515/med-2016-0055.

First Nations Studies Program. 2009. "Sixties Scoop." University of British Columbia, First Nations and Indigenous Studies. https://indigenous-foundations.arts.ubc.ca/sixties_scoop/.

Fleischmann, Robert, Julian Duhm, Hagen Hupperts, and Stephan A. Brandt. 2015. "Tablet Computers with Mobile Electronic Medical Records Enhance Clinical Routine and Promote Bedside Time: A Controlled Prospective Crossover Study." *Journal of Neurology* 262 (3): 532–40. doi: 10.1007/s00415-014-7581-7.

Folke, Carl 2006. "Resilience: The Emergence of a Perspective for Social-Ecological Systems Analyses." *Global Environmental Change* 16:253–67.

Folke, Carl, Thomas Hahn, Per Olsson, and Jon Norberg. 2005. "Adaptive Governance of Social-Ecological Systems." *Annual Review of Environment and Resources* 30:441–73.

Folkman, Susan, and Steven Greer. 2000. "Promoting Psychological Well-Being in the Face of Serious Illness: When Theory, Research and Practice Inform Each Other." *Psychooncology* 9:11–19.

Foster, Sam 2017. "Compassionate Leadership Counts." *British Journal of Nursing* 26 (12): 715. doi: 10.12968/bjon.2017.26.12.715.

Foucault, Michel. *The Birth of the Clinic: An Archaeology of Medical Perception.* Translated by Alan Sheridan. East Sussex: Psychology Press, 2003.

Frank, Arthur W. 2004. *The Renewal of Generosity: Illness, Medicine, and How to Live.* Chicago: University of Chicago Press.

– 2013. *The Wounded Storyteller: Body, Illness, and Ethics.* Chicago: University of Chicago Press.

Frank, Jason R., and Deborah Danoff. 2007. "The CanMEDS Initiative: Implementing an Outcomes-Based Framework of Physician Competencies." *Med Teach* 29 (7): 642–7. doi: 10.1080/01421590701746983.

Frank, Jason R., Mona Jabbour, and Peter Tugwell. 1996. "Skills for the New Millenium: Report of the Societal Needs Working Group, CanMEDS 2000 Project." *Annals Royal College of Physicians and Surgeons Canada* 29:209–16.

Franklin, Ursula. 1999. *The Real World of Technology.* Revised edition. CBC Massey Lectures Series. Toronto: House of Anansi Press.

Freeman, Steven F., Larry Hirschorn, and Marc David Maltz. 2004. "The Power of Moral Purpose: Sandler O'Neill & Partners in the Aftermath of September 11, 2001." *Ogranization Development Journal* 22 (4): 69–79.

Freire, Paulo. 2000. *Pedagogy of the Oppressed.* New York: Bloomsbury Publishing.

Frenk, Julio, Lincoln Chen, Zulfiqar A. Bhutta, Jordan Cohen, Nigel Crisp, Timothy Evans, Harvey Fineberg, et al. 2010. "Health Professionals for a New Century: Transforming Education to Strengthen Health Systems in an Interdependent World." *Lancet* 376 (9756): 1923–58. doi: 10.1016/s0140-6736(10)61854-5.

Gallop, Ruth, Patricia McKeever, Brenda Toner, William Lancee, and Marla Lueck. 1995. "The Impact of Childhood Sexual Abuse on the Psychological Well-Being and Practice of Nurses." *Archives of Psychiatric Nursing* 9 (3): 137–45.

Gardner, William L., Bruce J. Avolio, Fred Luthans, Douglas R. May, and Fred O. Walumbwa. 2005. "Can You See the Real Me? A Self-Based Model of Authentic Leader and Follower Development." *The Leadership Quarterly* 16 (3): 343–72.

Garg, Anmol, Rahul Singhal, Ved Ratn Dixit, and Astha Agarwal. n.d. "Artificial Emotional Intelligence." https://www.academia.edu/9830130/Artificial_Emotional_Intelligence.

Gates, Bill. 2013. "Here's My Plan to Improve Our World – and How You Can Help." *Wired*, 12 November 2013.

Gawande, Atul. 2018a. "The Upgrade." *New Yorker*, 12 November 2018, 62–72.

Gawande, Atul. 2018b. "Why Doctors Hate Their Computers." *New Yorker*, 5 November 2018, n.p.

Gilbert, Leah K., Matthew J. Breiding, Melissa T. Merrick, William W. Thompson, Derek C. Ford, Satvinder S. Dhingra, and Sharyn E. Parks. 2015. "Childhood Adversity and Adult Chronic Disease: An Update from Ten States and the District of Columbia, 2010." *Am J Prev Med* 48 (3): 345–9. doi: 10.1016/j.amepre.2014.09.006.

Gillan, Caitlin, Nicole Harnett, Emily Milne, Tom Purdie, David Wiljer, David Jaffray, and Brian Hodges. 2018. "Professional Implications of Introducing Artificial Intelligence in Healthcare: An Evaluation Using Radiation Medicine as a Testing Ground." *Journal of Medical Imaging and Radiation Sciences* 49 (1): S1–S2. doi: 10.1016/j.jmir.2018.02.006.

Goetz, Jennifer L., Dacher Keltner, and Emiliana Simon-Thomas. 2010. "Compassion: An Evolutionary Analysis and Empirical Review." *Psychological Bulletin* 136 (3): 351.

Goetz, Jennifer L., and Emiliana Simon-Thomas. 2017. "The Landscape of Compassion: Definitions and Scientific Approaches." In *The Oxford Handbook of Compassion Science*, edited by Emma M. Seppälä, Emiliana Simon-Thomas, Stephanie L. Brown, Monica C. Worline, C. Daryl Cameron, and Jame R. Doty, 3–15. New York: Oxford University Press.

Goldsmith, Marshall, and Mark Reiter. 2007. *What Got You Here Won't Get You There [How Successful People Become Even More Successful!]*. Sound recording. New York: Random House Audio.

Grant, Anthony M., Ingrid Studholme, Raj Verma, Lea Kirkwood, Bronwyn Paton, and Sean O'Connor. 2017. "The Impact of Leadership Coaching in an Australian Healthcare Setting." *Journal of Health Organization and Management* 31 (2): 237–52. doi: 10.1108/JHOM-09-2016-0187.

Greenleaf, Robert K. 1970. *The Servant as Leader*. Cambridge, MA: Center for Applied Studies.

Griffin, Ashley, Asheley Skinner, Jonathan Thornhill, and Morris Weinberger. 2016. "Patient Portals: Who Uses Them? What Features Do They Use?

And Do They Reduce Hospital Readmissions?" *Applied Clinical Informatics* 7 (2): 489–501. doi: 10.4338/ACI-2016-01-RA-0003.

Guille, Constance, Zhuo Zhao, John Krystal, Breck Nichols, Kathleen Brady, and Srijan Sen. 2015. "Web-Based Cognitive Behavioral Therapy Intervention for the Prevention of Suicidal Ideation in Medical Interns: A Randomized Clinical Trial." *JAMA Psychiatry* 72 (12): 1192–8. doi: 10.1001/jamapsychiatry.2015.1880.

Guo, Yan, Zhimeng Xu, Jiaying Qiao, Y. Alicia Hong, Hanxi Zhang, Chengbo Zeng, Weiping Cai, Linghua Li, and Cong Liu. 2018. "Development and Feasibility Testing of an mHealth (Text Message and WeChat) Intervention to Improve the Medication Adherence and Quality of Life of People Living with HIV in China: Pilot Randomized Controlled Trial." *JMIR mHealth and uHealth* 6 (9): e10274. doi: 10.2196/10274.

Hafferty, Frederick. W., and Donald W. Light. 1995. "Professional Dynamics and the Changing Nature of Medical Work." *Journal of Health and Social Behavior* Spec No:132–53.

Halbesleben, Jonathon R.B. 2006. "Sources of Social Support and Burnout: A Meta-analytic Test of the Conservation of Resources Model." *J Appl Psychol* 91 (5): 1134–45. doi: 10.1037/0021-9010.91.5.1134.

Hall, Louise H., Judith Johnson, Ian Watt, Anastasia Tsipa, and Daryl B. O'Connor. 2016. "Healthcare Staff Wellbeing, Burnout, and Patient Safety: A Systematic Review." *PLoS One* 11 (7): e0159015. doi: 10.1371/journal.pone.0159015.

Halman, Mark, Lindsay Baker, and Stella Ng. 2017. "Using Critical Consciousness to Inform Health Professions Education: A Literature Review." *Perspectives on Medical Education* 6 (1): 12–20. doi: 10.1007/s40037-016-0324-y.

Halpern, Janice, Robert G. Maunder, Brian Schwartz, and Maria Gurevich. 2012. "Attachment Insecurity, Responses to Critical Incident Distress, and Current Emotional Symptoms in Ambulance Workers." *Stress and Health* 28 (1): 51–60.

Hamel, Gary, and Liisa Välikangas. 2003. "The Quest for Resilience." *Harv. Bus. Rev* 81 (9): 52–63, 131.

Haque, Omar Sultan, and Adam Waytz. 2012. "Dehumanization in Medicine: Causes, Solutions, and Functions." *Perspectives on Psychological Science: A Journal of the Association for Psychological Science* 7 (2): 176–86. doi: 10.1177/1745691611429706.

Haraway, Donna. 1991. "Cyborg Manifesto: Science, Technology, and Socialist-Feminism in the Late Twentieth Century." In *Simians,*

Cyborgs and Women: The Reinvention of Nature, 149–181. New York: Routledge.

– 1988. "Situated Knowledges: The Science Question in Feminism and the Privilege of Partial Perspective." *Feminist Studies* 14 (3): 575–99.

Harding, Sandra. 1992. "Rethinking Standpoint Epistemology: What Is 'Strong Objectivity?'" *The Centennial Review* 36 (3): 437–70.

Hardy, Pip, and Tony Sumner. 2018. *Cultivating Compassion: How Digital Storytelling is Transforming Healthcare*. New York: Springer.

Hartrick Doane, Gweneth, and Colleen Varcoe. 2015. *How to Nurse: Relational Inquiry with Individuals and Families in Changing Health and Health Care Contexts*. New York: Wolters Kluwer Health/ Lippincott Williams & Wilkins.

Hawthornthwaite, Lisa, Taylor Roebotham, Lauren Lee, Mim O'Dowda, and Lorelei Lingard. 2018. "Three Sides to Every Story: Preparing Patient and Family Storytellers, Facilitators, and Audiences." *The Permanente Journal* 22: 17–119. doi: 10.7812/TPP/17-119.

HealthIt.gov. 2015. "What is a Patient Portal?" Office of the National Coordinator for Health Information Technology (website). www. healthit.gov/faq/what-patient-portal.

Hengstler, Monika, Ellen Enkel, and Selina Duelli. 2016. "Applied Artificial Intelligence and Trust – The Case of Autonomous Vehicles and Medical Assistance Devices." *Technological Forecasting and Social Change* 105:105–20. doi: 10.1016/j.techfore.2015.12.014.

Herbst, Anna M., Diane I. Swengros, and Gwen Kinney. 2010. "How to Teach Human Caring: Nurse Educator Role in Transformational Learning for a Large Healthcare System." *Journal for Nurses in Professional Development* 26 (4): E6–E11.

Hiles Howard, Amanda R., Sheri Parris, Jordan S. Hall, Casey D. Call, Erin Becker Razuri, Karyn B. Purvis, and David R. Cross. 2015. "An Examination of the Relationships between Professional Quality of Life, Adverse Childhood Experiences, Resilience, and Work Environment in a Sample of Human Service Providers." *Children and Youth Services Review* 57:141–8.

HIMSS Analytics. 2017. "The EMR Adoption Model." https://www. himssanalytics.org/emram.

Hoch, Dan, and Tom Ferguson. 2005. "What I've Learned from E-patients." *PLoS medicine* 2 (8):e206.

Hodges, Brian D. 2018. "Learning from Dorothy Vaughan: Artificial Intelligence and the Health Professions." *Medical Education* 52 (1): 11–13.

Hofmeyer, Anne, Luisa Toffoli, Rachael Vernon, Ruth Taylor, Hester C. Klopper, Siedine Knobloch Coetzee, and Dorrie Fontaine. 2018. "Teaching Compassionate Care to Nursing Students in a Digital Learning and Teaching Environment." *Collegian* 25 (3): 307–12.

Holden, Richard J. 2012. "Social and Personal Normative Influences on Healthcare Professionals to Use Information Technology: Towards a More Robust Social Ergonomics." *Theoretical Issues in Ergonomics Science* 13 (5): 546–69.

Holland, John H. 1998. *Emergence: From Chaos to Order*. Redwood City, CA: Addison-Wesley.

Holt-Lunstad, Julianne, Timothy B. Smith, Mark Baker, Tyler Harris, and David Stephenson. 2015. "Loneliness and Social Isolation as Risk Factors for Mortality: A Meta-analytic Review." *Perspectives on Psychological Science* 10 (2): 227–37.

Hooper, Crystal, Janet Craig, David. R. Janvrin, Margaret A. Wetsel, and Elaine Reimels. 2010. "Compassion Satisfaction, Burnout, and Compassion Fatigue among Emergency Nurses Compared with Nurses in Other Selected Inpatient Specialties." *J Emerg Nurs* 36 (5): 420–7. doi: 10.1016/j.jen.2009.11.027.

Hornett, Melanie. 2012. "Compassionate Leadership." *British Journal of Nursing* 21 (13): 831. doi: 10.12968/bjon.2012.21.13.831.

Hymel, Pamela A., Ronald R. Loeppke, Catherine M. Baase, Wayne N. Burton, Natalie P. Hartenbaum, T. Warner Hudson, Robert K. McLellan, et al. 2011. "Workplace Health Protection and Promotion: A New Pathway for a Healthier – and Safer – Workforce." *Journal of Occupational and Environmental Medicine* 53 (6): 695–702. doi: 10.1097/JOM.0b013e31822005do.

Institute for Safe Medication Practices. 2004. "Intimidation: Practitioners Speak Up about This Unresolved Problem." www.ismp.org/resources/intimidation-practitioners-speak-about-unresolved-problem-part-i.

Issacs, William. 1999. *Dialogue and the Art of Thinking Together*. New York: Random House.

Jaworski, Joseph. 2012. *Source: The Inner Path of Knowledge Creation*. Oakland, CA: Berrett-Koehler Publishers, Inc.

Johannesen, Jennifer. 2011. *No Ordinary Boy: The Life and Death of Owen Turney*. Toronto: Low to the Ground Pub.

John, Judith. 2016. *Convocation Speech: The Michener Institute of Education*. Toronto. https://www.youtube.com/watch?v=jJ3Re8a1ouo.

Johnson, Stephen. 2018. "In 1983, Isaac Asimov Predicted the World of 2019. Here's What He Got Right (and Wrong)." Big Think (website).

Jonah, Leigh, Annie-Claude Bourgeois, M. Edmunds, Amnan Awan,Olivia Varsaneux, and Winnie Siu. 2017. "AIDS in Canada-Surveillance Report, 2016." *Canada Communicable Disease Report* 43 (12): 257–61.

Jones, Jenny, Sarah Winch, Petra Strube, Marion Mitchell, and Amanda Henderson. 2016. "Delivering Compassionate Care in Intensive Care Units: Nurses' Perceptions of Enablers and Barriers." *Journal of Advanced Nursing* 72 (12): 3137–46. doi: 10.1111/jan.13064.

Jong, Michael, Ivar Mendez, and Robert Jong. 2019. "Enhancing Access to Care in Northern Rural Communities via Telehealth." *International Journal of Circumpolar Health* 78 (2):1554174. doi: 10.1080/ 22423982.2018.1554174.

Jung, Carl G. 1928. *Contributions to Analytical Psychology, International Library of Psychology, Philosophy, and Scientific Method*. London: K. Paul, Trench, Trubner & Co.

Kabat-Zinn, Jon. 2016. *Midnfulness for Beginners: Reclaiming the Present Moment – and Your Life*. Boulder, CO: Sounds True.

Kahn, Marc J., Ralph Maurer, Steven A. Wartman, and Benjamin P. Sachs. 2014. "A Case for Change: Disruption in Academic Medicine." *Acad Med* 89 (9): 1216–19. doi: 10.1097/ACM.0000000000000418.

Kanov, Jason M., Sally Maitlis, Monica C. Worline, Jane E. Dutton, Peter J. Frost, and Jacoba M. Lilius. 2004. "Compassion in Organizational Life." *American Behavioral Scientist* 47 (6): 808–27. doi: 10.1177/ 0002764203260211.

Keasberry, Justin, Ian A. Scott, Clair Sullivan, Andrew Staib, and Richard Ashby. 2018. "Going Digital: A Narrative Overview of the Clinical and Organisational Impacts of eHealth Technologies in Hospital Practice." *Australian Health Review* 41 (6): 646–64.

Kemp, Jessica, Timothy Zhang, Fiona Inglis, David Wiljer, Sanjeev Sockalingam, Allison Crawford, Brian Lo, et al. 2020. "Delivery of Compassionate Mental Health Care in a Digital Technology-Driven Age: Scoping Review." *Journal of Medical Internet Research* 22 (3): e16263 doi: 10.2196/16263.

Kendall, Claire E., Esther S. Shoemaker, Janet Raboud, Amy E. Mark, Ahmed M. Bayoumi, Ann N. Burchell, Mona Loutfy, Sean B. Rourke, Clare E. Liddy, and Ron. Rosenes. 2018. "Assessing Timely Presentation to Care among People Diagnosed with HIV during Hospital Admission: A Population-Based Study in Ontario, Canada." *AIDS and Behavior*:1–9.

Khan, Ibrahim, Nnamdi Ndubuka, Kris Stewart, Veronica. McKinney, and Ivar Mendez. 2017. "The Use of Technology to Iimprove Health Care to

Saskatchewan's First Nations Communities." *Canada Communicable Disease Report* 43 (6): 120–4.

King, Elizabeth, Karen Kinvig, Jonathan Steif, Annie Q. Qiu, Evelyn J. Maan, Arianne Y.K. Albert, Neora Pick, et al. 2017. "Mobile Text Messaging to Improve Medication Adherence and Viral Load in a Vulnerable Canadian Population Living with Human Immunodeficiency Virus: A Repeated Measures Study." *Journal of Medical Internet Research* 19 (6): e190. doi: 10.2196/jmir.6631.

Kingsley, Patrick, and Safak Timur. 2015. "Stories of 2015: How Alan Kurdi's Death Changed the World." *Guardian*, 31 December 2015.

Kivimaki, Mika, Marko Elovainio, Jussi Vahtera, and Jane E. Ferrie. 2003. "Organisational Justice and Health of Employees: Prospective Cohort Study." *Occup Environ Med* 60 (1): 27–33; discussion 33–4.

Kohane, Isaac. 2018. "The Beauty of 'Small Data' in Medicine, from Measuring Kids to Tumor Mutations." *CommonHealth*, 29 August 2018.

Krakovsky, Marina. 2018. "Artificial (Emotional) Intelligence." *Communications of the ACM* 61 (4): 18–19.

Krasner, Michael S., Ronald M. Epstein, Howard Beckman, Anthony L. Suchman, Benjamin Chapman, Christopher J. Mooney, and Timothy E. Quill. 2009. "Association of an Educational Program in Mindful Communication with Burnout, Empathy, and Attitudes among Primary Care Physicians." *JAMA* 302 (12): 1284–93. doi: 10.1001/jama.2009.1384.

Kruse, Clemens Scott, Benjamin Frederick, Taylor Jacobson, and D. Kyle Monticone. 2017. "Cybersecurity in Healthcare: A Systematic Review of Modern Threats and Trends." *Technology and Health Care* 25 (1): 1–10.

Kumagai, Arno K., and Thirusha Naidu. 2015. "Reflection, Dialogue, and the Possibilities of Space." *Academic Medicine* 90 (3): 283–8.

Kuper, Ayelet. 2016. "When I Say … Equity." *Medical Education* 50 (3): 283–4. doi: doi:10.1111/medu.12954.

Kuper, Ayelet, Scott Reeves, Mathieu Albert, and Brian David Hodges. 2007. "Assessment: Do We Need to Broaden Our Methodological Horizons?" *Medical Education* 41 (12): 1121–3.

Landy, Rachel, Cathy Cameron, Anson Au, Debra Cameron, Kelly O'Brien, Katherine Robrigado, Larry Baxter, Lynn Cockburn, Shawna O'Hearn, and Brent Olivier. "Educational Strategies to Enhance Reflexivity among Clinicians and Health Professional Students: A Scoping Study." 2016.

Lane, Christopher. 2018. "Digital Health and the Rise of Mental Health Apps." *Psychology Today* (website). 11 August.

Lanier, Cédric, Melissa Dominicé Dao, Patricia Hudelson, Bernard Cerutti, and Noëlle Junod Perron. 2017. "Learning to Use Electronic Health Records: Can We Stay Patient-Centered? A Pre-post Intervention Study with Family Medicine Residents." *BMC Family Practice* 18 (1): 1–11. doi: 10.1186/s12875-017-0640-2.

Laschinger, Heather K., Joan Almost, and Donnalene Tuer-Hodes. 2003. "Workplace Empowerment and Magnet Hospital Characteristics: Making the Link." *J Nurs Adm* 33 (7–8): 410–22.

Lashbrook, Angela. 2018. "AI-Driven Dermatology Could Leave Dark-Skinned Patients Behind." *The Atlantic* (website). 16 August.

Lee, SooJong, Joung H. Lee, Marion Gillen, and Niklas Krause. 2014. "Job Stress and Work-Related Musculoskeletal Symptoms among Intensive Care Unit Nurses: A Comparison between Job Demand-Control and Effort-Reward Imbalance Models." *Am J Ind Med* 57 (2): 214–21. doi: 10.1002/ajim.22274.

Lemaire, Jane B., Jean E. Wallace, Kelly Dinsmore, and Delia Roberts. 2011. "Food for Thought: An Exploratory Study of How Physicians Experience Poor Workplace Nutrition." *Nutrition Journal* 10 (1): 18. doi: 10.1186/1475-2891-10-18.

Lester, Richard T., Paul Ritvo, Edward J. Mills, Antony Kariri, Sarah Karanja, Michael H. Chung, William Jack, James Habyarimana, Mohsen Sadatsafavi, and Mehdi Najafzadeh. 2010. "Effects of a Mobile Phone Short Message Service on Antiretroviral Treatment Adherence in Kenya (WelTel Kenya1): A Randomised Trial." *Lancet* 376 (9755): 1838–45.

Lexico. 2020. "Metacognition." Lexico.com (website). Oxford University Press. https://www.lexico.com/en/definition/metacognition.

Li, David, Kulamakan Kulasegaram, and Brian D. Hodges. 2019. "Why We Needn't Fear the Machines: Opportunities for Medicine in a Machine Learning World." *Acad Med* 94 (5): 623–5. doi: 10.1097/ACM.0000000000002661.

Linzer, Mark, Sara Poplau, Ellie Grossman, Anita Varkey, Steven Yale, Eric Williams, Lanis Hicks, et al. 2015. "A Cluster Randomized Trial of Interventions to Improve Work Conditions and Clinician Burnout in Primary Care: Results from the Healthy Work Place (HWP) Study." *J Gen Intern Med* 30 (8): 1105–11. doi: 10.1007/s11606-015-3235-4.

Lu, Dave W., Paul L. Weygandt, Carrie Pinchbeck, and Tania D. Strout. 2018. "Emergency Medicine Trainee Burnout Is Associated With Lower Patients' Satisfaction with Their Emergency Department Care." *AEM Educ Train* 2 (2): 86–90. doi: 10.1002/aet2.10094.

Lucas, Brian P., William E. Trick, Arthur T. Evans, Benjamin Mba, Jennifer
    Smith, Krishna Das, Peter Clarke, Anita Varkey, Suja Mathew, and
    Robert A. Weinstein. 2012. "Effects of 2- vs 4-week Attending Physician
    Inpatient Rotations on Unplanned Patient Revisits, Evaluations by
    Trainees, and Attending Physician Burnout: A Randomized Trial."
    JAMA 308 (21): 2199–207. doi: 10.1001/jama.2012.36522.
Lukes, Steven. 2005. *Power: A Radical View*. 2nd ed. New York: Palgrave
    MacMillan.
Lynch, Jamie. 2017. "The Worst Computer Bugs in History: Race
    conditions in Therac-25." *Bugsnag* (blog), 19 September. https://www.
    bugsnag.com/blog/bug-day-race-condition-therac-25.
Makadia, Rakhee, Rachel Sabin-Farrell, and Graham Turpin. 2017.
    "Indirect Exposure to Client Trauma and the Impact on Trainee Clinical
    Psychologists: Secondary Traumatic Stress or Vicarious
    Traumatization?" *Clin Psychol Psychother* 24 (5): 1059–68. doi:
    10.1002/cpp.2068.
Mallette, Claire, Don Rose, Karen Poole, Carolyn Byrne, and Alice
    Ormiston. 2018. *AMS Phoenix Project grant report: Exploring caring
    in Nursing Curricula in Ontario, a Provincial Nursing Education
    Initiative*. Toronto: Ontario.
Marine, Albert, Jani Ruotsalainen, Consol Serra, and Jos Verbeek. 2006.
    "Preventing Occupational Stress in Healthcare Workers." *Cochrane
    Database Syst Rev* (4): CD002892. doi: 10.1002/14651858.CD002892.
    pub2.
Marmot, Michael. 2015. *The Health Gap: The Challenge of an Unequal
    World*. New York: Bloomsbury.
Marmot, Michael G., George.D. Smith, S. Stansfeld, C. Patel, F. North, J.
    Head, I. White, E. Brunner, and A. Feeney. 1991. "Health Inequalities
    among British Civil Servants: The Whitehall II Study." *Lancet* 337
    (8754): 1387–93.
Martimianakis, Maria Athina, and Frederic W. Hafferty. 2016. "Exploring
    the Interstitial Space between the Ideal and the Practised: Humanism
    and the Hidden Curriculum of System Reform." *Medical Education*
    50 (3): 278–80. doi: 10.1111/medu.12982.
Maslach, Christina, Susan E. Jackson, and Michael P. Leitner. 1997.
    "Maslach Burnout Inventory: Third edition." In *Evaluating Stress:
    A Book of Resources*, edited by Carlos P. Zalaquett and Richard J.
    Wood, 191–218. Lanham, MD: Scarecrow Press.
Maunder, Robert G., Janice Halpern, Brian Schwartz, and Maria
    Gurevich. 2012. "Symptoms and Responses to Critical Incidents

in Paramedics who Have Experienced Childhood Abuse and Neglect." *Emerg Med J* 29 (3): 222–7. doi: 10.1136/emj.2010.099838.

Maunder, Robert G., and Jonathan J. Hunter. 2001. "Attachment and Psychosomatic Medicine: Developmental Contributions to Stress and Disease." *Psychosomatic Med* 63 (4): 556–67.

Maunder, Robert G., and Jonathan Hunter. 2015. *Love, Fear, and Health: How Our Attachments to Others Shape Health and Health Care.* Toronto: University of Toronto Press.

Maunder, Robert G., Jonathan Hunter, Leslie Vincent, Jocelyn Bennett, Nathalie Peladeau, Molyn Leszcz, Joel Sadavoy, Lieve M. Verhaeghe, Rosalie Steinberg, and Tony Mazzulli. 2003. "The Immediate Psychological and Occupational Impact of the 2003 SARS Outbreak in a Teaching Hospital." *CMAJ* 168 (10): 1245–51.

Maunder, Robert G., Jonathan J. Hunter, and William J. Lancee. 2011. "The Impact of Attachment Insecurity and Sleep Disturbance on Symptoms and Sick Days in Hospital-Based Health-Care Workers." *J Psychosom Res* 70 (1): 11–17.

Maunder, Robert G., William J. Lancee, Kenneth E. Balderson, Jocelyn P. Bennett, Bjug Borgundvaag, Susan Evans, Christopher Fernandes, et al. 2006. "Long-Term Psychological and Occupational Effects of Providing Hospital Healthcare during SARS Outbreak." *Emerging Infectious Diseases* 12:1924–32.

Maunder, Robert G., William J. Lancee, Reet Mae, Leslie Vincent, Nathalie Peladeau, Mary A. Beduz, Jonathan J. Hunter, and Molyn Leszcz. 2010. "Computer-Assisted Resilience Training to Prepare Healthcare Workers for Pandemic Influenza: A Randomized Trial of the Optimal Dose of Training." *BMC Health Serv. Res* 10:72. https://doi.org/10.1186/1472-6963-10-72.

Maunder, Robert G., William J. Lancee, Sean B. Rourke, Jonathan Hunter, David S. Goldbloom, Patricia M. Petryshen, Molyn Leszcz, et al. 2005. "The Experience of the 2003 SARS Outbreak as a Traumatic Stress among Frontline Healthcare Workers in Toronto: Lessons Learned." In *SARS: A Case Study in Emerging Infections*, edited by Angeal R. McLean, Robert M. May, John Pattison and Robin A. Weiss, 96–106. Oxford: Oxford University Press.

Maunder, Robert G., Molyn Leszcz, David Savage, Mary A. Adam, Nathalie Peladeau, Donna Romano, Marci Rose, and Bernard Schulman. 2008. "Applying the Lessons of SARS to Pandemic Influenza: An Evidence-Based Approach to Mitigating the Stress Experienced by Healthcare Workers." *Can J Public Health* 99 (6): 486–8.

Maunder, Robert G., Nathalie Peladeau, David Savage, and William J.
Lancee. 2010. "The Prevalence of Childhood Adversity among
Healthcare Workers and its Relationship to Adult Life Events,
Distress and Impairment." *Child Abuse Negl* 34 (2): 114–23.

McCabe, Catherine, and Fiona Timmins. 2016. "Embracing Healthcare
Technology – What Is the Way Forward for Nurse Education?" *Nurse
Education in Practice* 21:104–6.

McClure, Margaret, Muriel Poulin, and Margaret D. Sovie. 1983.
"Magnet Hospitals: Attraction and Retention of Professional Nurses."
American Academy of Nursing, Kansas City, MO.

McConnell, Meghan M., and Kevin W. Eva. 2012. "The Role of Emotion
in the Learning and Transfer of Clinical Skills and Knowledge."
*Academic Medicine: Journal of the Association of American Medical
Colleges* 87 (10): 1316–22. doi: 10.1097/ACM.0b013e3182675af2.

Mental Health Commission of Canada. 2017. *Addressing the Access
Gap: Leveraging the Potential of eMental Health in Canada.*
Vancouver, BC.

Merriam-Webster. 2004. "Technology." *Merriam-Webster's Collegiate
Dictionary (11th ed.):* Springfield: Merriam-Webster Incorporated.

Meskó, Bertalan, Zsófia Drobni, Éva Bényei, Bence Gergely, and
Zsuzsanna Győrffy. 2017. "Digital Health Is a Cultural Transformation
of Traditional Healthcare." *mHealth* 3:38.

Mezirow, Jack. 1991. *Transformative Dimensions of Adult Learning.*
1st ed., The Jossey-Bass Higher and Adult Education series. San
Francisco: Jossey-Bass.

Mickan, Sharon, Helen Atherton, Nia W. Roberts, Carl Heneghan, and
Julie K. Tilson. 2014. "Use of Handheld Computers in Clinical Practice:
A Systematic Review." *BMC Medical Informatics and Decision Making*
14 (56). doi: 10.1186/1472-6947-14-56.

Mignolo, Walter D., and Catherine E. Walsh. 2018. *On Decoloniality:
Concepts, Analytics, and Praxis.* Durham, NC: Duke University Press.

Mogoba, Phepo, Tamsin K. Phillips, Landon Myer, Linda Ndlovu,
Martin C. Were, and Kate Clouse. 2019. "Smartphone Usage and
Preferences among Postpartum HIV-positive Women in South Africa."
AIDS care: 1–7.

Monsalve-Reyes, Carlos S., Concepción San Luis-Costas, Jose L. Gomez-
Urquiza, Luis Albendín-García, Raimundo Aguayo, and Guillermo A.
Canadas-De la Fuente. 2018. "Burnout Syndrome and Its Prevalence
in Primary Care Nursing: A Systematic Review and Meta-analysis."
BMC Fam Pract 19 (59). doi: 10.1186/s12875-018-0748-z.

Montgomery, Kathryn, Jeff Chester, and Katharina Kopp. 2018. "Health
    Wearables: Ensuring Fairness, Preventing Discrimination, and Promoting
    Equity in an Emerging Internet-of-Things Environment." *Journal of
    Information Policy* 8:34–77. doi: 10.5325/jinfopoli.8.2018.0034.
MSI (Minority Serving Institutions). 2013. "Substance Abuse and Mental
    Health Services Administration." https://www.samhsa.gov/sites/default/
    files/grants/pdf/sp-14-005_0.pdf.
Murray, Elizabeth. 2014. "eHealth: Where Next?" *Br J Gen Pract*. vol. 64
    (624): 325–6.
Mylod, Deirdre E., and Thomas H. Lee. "Framework for Reducing
    Suffering in Health Care." *Harvard Business Review*. 14 November.
    Accessed 17 December 2018. https://hbr.org/2013/11/a-framework-
    for-reducing-suffering-in-health-care.
Naidu, Thirusha, and Arno K. Kumagai. 2016. "Troubling Muddy Waters:
    Problematizing Reflective Practice in Global Medical Education."
    Academic Medicine 91 (3): 317–21.
Ndofirepi, Amasa Philip, and Ephraim Taurai Gwaravanda. 2018.
    "Epistemic (In)justice in African Universities: A Perspective of the
    Politics of Knowledge." *Educational Review*:1–14. doi: 10.1080/
    00131911.2018.1459477.
Needleman, Jack. 2013. "Increasing Acuity, Increasing Technology, and
    the Changing Demands on Nurses." *Nursing economic$* 31 (4): 200–2.
Neufeld, Vic R., Robert F. Maudsley, Richard J. Pickering, B.C. Walters,
    Jeffrey M. Turnbull, Robert A. Spasoff, David J. Hollomby, and
    K.J. LaVigne. 1993. "Demand-Side Medical Education: Educating
    Future Physicians for Ontario." *CMAJ* 148 (9): 1471–7.
Nguyen, Quoc Dinh, Nicolas Fernandez, Thierry Karsenti, and Bernard
    Charlin. 2014. "What Is Reflection? A Conceptual Analysis of Major
    Definitions and a Proposal of a Five-Component Model." *Medical
    Education* 48 (12): 1176–89.
Nishnawbe Aski Nation. 2019. "Health Transformation. Progress Report.
    Fall 2019." http://www.nan.on.ca/upload/documents/nan-ht-report-
    oct-28-2019.pdf.
Noble, Safiya Umoja. 2018. *Algorithms of Oppression: How Search
    Engines Reinforce Racism*. New York: NYU Press.
Oxford Paperback Dictionary. 2009. "Medicine." 3rd ed. New York:
    Oxford University Press.
O'Brien, Nadia, Saara Greene, Allison Carter, Johanna Lewis, Valerie
    Nicholson, Gladys Kwaramba, Brigitte Ménard, et al. 2017.
    "Envisioning Women-Centered HIV Care: Perspectives from Women

Living with HIV in Canada." *Women's Health Issues* 27 (6): 721–30. doi: 10.1016/j.whi.2017.08.001.

Ogilvie, Megan. 2020. "Your Next Visit with a Doctor May not be Face to Face. Ontario Shifting to Virtual First Model in a Bid to Halt Spread of COVID-19," *Star*, 16 March. https://www.thestar.com/news/gta/2020/03/16/your-next-visit-to-a-doctor-may-not-be-face-to-face-ontario-shifting-to-virtual-first-model-in-bid-to-halt-spread-of-covid-19.html.

Oh, Hans, Carlos Rizo, Murray Enkin, and Alejandro Jadad. 2005. "What Is eHealth (3): A Systematic Review of Published Definitions." *Journal of Medical Internet Research* 7 (1): e1.

Okun, Sally, and Christine A Caligtan. 2016. "The Engaged ePatient." *Health Informatics: An Interprofessional Approach* 2:204–19.

Oreskovich, Michael R., Krista L. Kaups, Charles M. Balch, John B. Hanks, Daneil Satele, Jeff Sloan, Charles Meredith, Amanda Buhl, Lotte N. Dyrbye, and Tait D. Shanafelt. 2012. "Prevalence of Alcohol Use Disorders among American Surgeons." *Arch Surg* 147 (2): 168–74. doi: 10.1001/archsurg.2011.1481.

Padilla Fortunatti, Cristobal, and Yasna K. Palmeiro-Silva. 2017. "Effort-Reward Imbalance and Burnout among ICU Nursing Staff: A Cross-Sectional Study." *Nurs Res* 66 (5): 410–16. doi: 10.1097/NNR.0000000000000239.

Panagioti, Maria, Keith Geraghty, Judith Johnson, Anil Zhou, Efharis Panagopoulou, Carolyn Chew-Graham, David Peters, Alexander Hodkinson, Ruth Riley, and Aneez Esmail. 2018. "Association between Physician Burnout and Patient Safety, Professionalism, and Patient Satisfaction: A Systematic Review and Meta-analysis." *JAMA Intern Med.* 178(10): 1317–31. doi: 10.1001/jamainternmed.2018.3713.

Panagioti, Maria, Efharis Panagopoulou, Peter Bower, George Lewith, Evangelis Kontopantelis, Carolyn Chew-Graham, Shoba Dawson, Harm van Marwijk, Keith Geraghty, and Aneez Esmail. 2017. "Controlled Interventions to Reduce Burnout in Physicians: A Systematic Review and Meta-analysis." *JAMA Intern Med* 177 (2): 195–205. doi: 10.1001/jamainternmed.2016.7674.

Panagiotou, Irene, Stelios Katsaragakis, Eleni Tsilika, and Efi Parpa. 2009. "Ethical and Practical Challenges in Implementing Informed Consent in HIV/AIDS Clinical Trials in Developing or Resource-Limited Countries." *SAHARA-J: Journal of Social Aspects of HIV/AIDS* 6 (2): 46–57. doi: 10.1080/17290376.2009.9724930.

Parshuram, Christopher S., Andre C. Amaral, Niall D. Ferguson, G. Ross Baker, Edward E. Etchells, Virginia Flintoft, John Granton, et al. 2015.

"Patient Safety, Resident Well-Being and Continuity of Care with Different Resident Duty Schedules in the Intensive Care Unit: A Randomized Trial." *CMAJ* 187 (5): 321–9. doi: 10.1503/cmaj.140752.

Pattani, Reena, Shiphra Ginsburg, Alekhya Mascarenhas Johnson, Julia E. Moore, Sabrina Jassemi, and Sharon E. Straus. 2018. "Organizational Factors Contributing to Incivility at an Academic Medical Center and Systems-Based Solutions: A Qualitative Study." *Academic Medicine* 93 (10): 1569–75. doi: 10.1097/ACM.0000000000002310.

Patton, Michael Quinn. 2010. *Developmental Evaluation: Applying Complexity Concepts to Enhance Innovation and Use.* New York: Guilford Press.

"Pepper-Uppers – Japan is Embracing Nursing Care Robots." *The Economist,* 25 November 2017, 60–1. https://www.economist.com/news/business/21731677-around-5000-nursing-care-homes-across-country-are-testing-robots-japan-embracing.

Pfuntner, Anne, Lauren M. Wier, and Carolyn Stocks. 2013. "Most Frequent Conditions in U.S. Hospitals, 2011: Statistical Brief #162." In *Healthcare Cost and Utilization Project (HCUP) Statistical Briefs.* Rockville (MD).

Philpott, Jane. 2018. "Canada's Efforts to Ensure the Health and Wellbeing of Indigenous Peoples." *Lancet* 391 (10131): 1650–1.

Porter, Michael E., and Elizabeth O. Teisberg. 2006. *Redefining Health Care: Creating Value-Based Competition on Results.* Boston: Harvard Business School Press.

Portoghese, Igor, Maura Galletta, Ross C. Coppola, Gabriele Finco, and Marcello Campagna. 2014. "Burnout and Workload among Health Care Workers: The Moderating Role of Job Control." *Saf Health Work* 5 (3): 152–7. doi: 10.1016/j.shaw.2014.05.004.

Powell, Philip A., and Jennifer Roberts. 2017. "Situational Determinants of Cognitive, Affective, and Compassionate Empathy in Naturalistic Digital Interactions." *Computers in Human Behavior* 68:137–48.

Powles, Julia, and Hal Hodson. 2017. "Google DeepMind and Healthcare in an Age of Algorithms." *Health and Technology* 7 (4): 351–67.

Ramage, Charlotte, Kathy Curtis, Angela Glynn, Julia Montgomery, Elona Hoover, Jane Leng, Clare Martin, Catherine Theodosius, and Ann Gallagher. 2017. "Developing and Using a Toolkit for Cultivating Compassion in Healthcare: An Appreciative Inquiry Approach." *International Journal of Practice-Based Learning in Health and Social Care* 5 (1): 42–64.

Rashotte, Judy, Lara Varpio, Kathy Day, Craig Kuziemsky, Avi Parush, Pat Elliott-Miller, James W. King, and Tyson Roffey. 2016. "Mapping

Communication Spaces: The Development and Use of a Tool for Analyzing the Impact of EHRs on Interprofessional Collaborative Practice." *International Journal of Medical Informatics* 93:2–13.

RBC (Royal Bank of Canada). 2018. "Humans Wanted: How Canadian Youth Can Thrive in the Age of Disruption." Royal Bank of Canada (website). www.rbc.com/dms/enterprise/futurelaunch/humans-wanted-how-canadian-youth-can-thrive-in-the-age-of-disruption.html.

Reay, Trish, and C.R. (Bob) Hinings. 2009. "Managing the Rivalry of Competing Institutional Logics." *Organization Studies* 30 (6): 629–52. doi: 10.1177/0170840609104803.

Richardson, Cliff, Marcus Percy, and Jane Hughes. 2015. "Nursing Therapeutics: Teaching Student Nurses Care, Compassion and Empathy." *Nurse Education Today* 35 (5): e1–e5.

Richardson, Lisa, and Tracy Murphy. 2018. *Bringing Reconciliation to Healthcare in Canada: Wise Practices for Healthcare Leaders*. Ottawa: HealthCareCAN.

Rimmer, Abi. 2014. "Why Do Female Doctors Earn Less Money for Doing the Same Job?" *BMJ* 349:g5604. doi: 10.1136/bmj.g5604.

Risling, Tracie. 2017. "Educating the Nurses of 2025: Technology Trends of the Next Decade." *Nurse Education in Practice* 22:89–92.

Rowland, Paula, Sarah E. McMillan, Maria A. Martimianakis, and Brian D. Hodges. 2018. "Learning from Patients: Constructions of Knowledge and Legitimacy in Hospital Based Quality Improvement Programs." *Studies in Continuing Education* 40 (3): 337–50. doi: 10.1080/0158037X.2018.1465402.

Said, Edward W. 1979. *Orientalism*. New York: Vintage Books.

Salyers, Michelle P., Kelsey A. Bonfils, Lauren Luther, Ruth L. Firmin, Dominique A. White, Erin L. Adams, and Angela L. Rollins. 2017. "The Relationship between Professional Burnout and Quality and Safety in Healthcare: A Meta-analysis." *J Gen Intern Med* 32 (4): 475–82. doi: 10.1007/s11606-016-3886-9.

Sanchez-Laws, Ana Luisa. 2010. "Digital Storytelling as an Emerging Documentary Form." *Seminar.net* 6(3). https://journals.hioa.no/index.php/seminar/article/view/2426.

Sarason, Seymour B. 1977. *Caring and Compassion in Clinical Practice: Issues in the Selection, Training, and Behavior of Helping Professionals*. 1st ed. Northvale, NJ: Jason Aronson, Inc.

Sardar, Ziauddin, ed. 1988. *The Revenge of Athena: Science, Exploitation and the Third World*. London: Mansell.

Scambler, Graham. 2009. "Health-Related Stigma." *Sociology of Health & Illness* 31 (3): 441–55. doi: 10.1111/j.1467-9566.2009.01161.x.

Schaink, Alexis Kerry, K. Kuluski, Renée F. Lyons, Martin Fortin, Alejandro R. Jadad, Ross Upshur, and Walter P. Wodchis. 2012. "A Scoping Review and Thematic Classification of Patient Complexity: Offering a Unifying Framework." *J Comorb* 2:1–9.

Scharmer, C. Otto. 2007a. "Addressing the Blind Spot of Our Time: An Executive Summary of the New Book by Otto Scharmer *Theory U: Leading from the Future as It Emerges*." The Presencing Institute.

Scharmer, Otto. 2007b. *Theory U: Leading from the Future as It Emerges*. Cambridge, MA: The Society for Organizational Learning.

Schoenwald, Sonja K., Kimberly Eaton Hoagwood, Marc S. Atkins, Mary E. Evans, and Heather Ringeisen. 2010. "Workforce Development and the Organization of Work: The Science We Need." *Administration and Policy in Mental Health* 37 (1–2): 71–80. doi: 10.1007/s10488-010-0278-z.

Seppälä, Emma M., Emiliana Simon-Thomas, Stephanie L. Brown, Monica C. Worline, C. Daryl Cameron, and James R. Doty. 2017. *The Oxford Handbook of Compassion Science*: Oxford University Press.

Serhal, Eva, Amanda Arena, Sanjeev Sockalingam, Linda Mohri, and Allison Crawford. 2018. "Adapting the Consolidated Framework for Implementation Research to Create Organizational Readiness and Implementation Tools for Project ECHO." *The Journal of Continuing Education in the Health Professions* 38 (2): 145.

Serhal, Eva, Allison Crawford, Joyce Cheng, and Paul Kurdyak. 2017. "Implementation and Utilisation of Telepsychiatry in Ontario: A Population-Based Study." *The Canadian Journal of Psychiatry* 62 (10): 716–25.

Sevean, Patricia, Sally Dampier, Michelle Spadoni, Shane Strickland, and Susan Pilatzke. 2008. "Bridging the Distance: Educating Nurses for Telehealth Practice." *The Journal of Continuing Education in Nursing* 39 (9): 413–18.

Sevunts, Levon. 2017. "Will Your Doctor Be Replaced by a Robot?" *Radio Canada International*, 10 May 2017.

Shachak, Aviv, Michael Hadas-Dayagi, Amitai Ziv, and Shmeul Reis. 2009. "Primary Care Physicians' Use of an Electronic Medical Record System: A Cognitive Task Analysis." *J Gen Intern Med* 24 (3): 341–8. doi: 10.1007/s11606-008-0892-6.

Shanafelt, Tait D. 2018. "Physician Burnout: Stop Blaming the Individual." *NEJM Catalyst*, accessed 5 September 2018. http://catalyst.nejm.org/videos/physician-burnout-stop-blaming-the-individual/.

Shanafelt, Tait D., Charles M. Balch, Lotte Dyrbye, Gerald Bechamps, Tom Russell, D. Satele, Teresa Rummans, et al. 2011. "Special Report:

Suicidal Ideation among American Surgeons." *Arch Surg* 146 (1): 54–62. doi: 10.1001/archsurg.2010.292.

Shanafelt, Tait D., Lotte N. Dyrbye, Christine Sinsky, Omar Hasan, Daniel Satele, Jeff Sloan, and Colin P. West. 2016. "Relationship between Clerical Burden and Characteristics of the Electronic Environment with Physician Burnout and Professional Satisfaction." *Mayo Clin Proc* 91 (7): 836–48. doi: 10.1016/j.mayocp.2016.05.007.

Shanafelt, Tait D., Lotte N. Dyrbye, and Colin P. West. 2017. "Addressing Physician Burnout: The Way Forward." *JAMA* 317 (9): 901–02. doi: 10.1001/jama.2017.0076.

Shanafelt, Tait D., Joel Goh, and Christine Sinsky. 2017. "The Business Case for Investing in Physician Well-Being." *JAMA Intern Med* 177 (12): 1826–32. doi: 10.1001/jamainternmed.2017.4340.

Shanafelt, Tait D., and John H. Noseworthy. 2017. "Executive Leadership and Physician Well-Being: Nine Organizational Strategies to Promote Engagement and Reduce Burnout." *Mayo Clin Proc* 92 (1): 129–46. doi: 10.1016/j.mayocp.2016.10.004.

Shanafelt, Tait D., Jeff A. Sloan, and Thomas M. Habermann. 2003. "The Well-Being of Physicians." *Am J Med* 114 (6): 513–9.

Shaw, Stacey. 2015. "The Psychology of Computer Rage." *Psychology In Action*, 27 September 2015. https://www.psychologyinaction.org/psychology-in-action-1/2015/12/27/the-psychology-of-computer-rage.

Shen, Nelson, Thérèse Bernier, Lydia Sequeira, John Strauss, Michelle Silver, Abigail Carter-Langford, and David Wiljer. 2019. "Understanding Patient Privacy Perspective on Health Information Exchange: A Systematic." *International Journal of Medical Informatics* 125 (May): 1–12.

Siegrist, J. 1996. "Adverse Health Effects of High-Effort/Low-Reward Conditions." *J Occup. Health Psychol* 1 (1): 27–41.

Sileo, Katelyn M., Rebecca Fielding-Miller, Shari L. Dworkin, and Paul J. Fleming. 2018. "What Role Do Masculine Norms Play in Men's HIV Testing in Sub-Saharan Africa? A Scoping Review." *AIDS and Behavior* 22 (8): 2468–79. doi: 10.1007/s10461-018-2160-z.

Sinclair, Helen A., and Conal Hamill. 2007. "Does Vicarious Traumatisation Affect Oncology Nurses? A Literature Review." *Eur J Oncol Nurs* 11 (4): 348–56. doi: 10.1016/j.ejon.2007.02.007.

Skloot, Rebecca. 2010. *The Immortal Life of Henrietta Lacks*. New York: Crown Publishers.

Skloot, Rebecca. 2013. "The Immortal Life of Henrietta Lacks, the Sequel." *New York Times*, 23 March.

Smith, Daryl G. 2012. "Building Institutional Capacity for Diversity and Inclusion in Academic Medicine." *Acad Med* 87 (11): 1511–15. doi: 10.1097/ACM.0b013e31826d30d5.

Smith, Linda Tuhiwai. 1999. *Decolonizing Methodologies: Research and Indigenous Peoples*. Winnipeg: Zed Books.

– 2008. "On Tricky Ground: Researching the Native in the Age of Uncertainty." In *The Landscape of Qualitative Research*, edited by Norman K. Denzin and Yvonna S. Lincoln, 85–113. Los Angeles: SAGE Publications.

Soares, Joaquim J., Giorgio Grossi, and Örjan Sundin. 2007. "Burnout among Women: Associations with Demographic/Socio-economic, Work, Life-Style and Health Factors." *Arch Womens Ment Health* 10 (2): 61–71. doi: 10.1007/s00737-007-0170-3.

Soler, Jean K., Hakan Yaman, Magdalena Esteva, Frank Dobbs, Radist S. Asenova, Milica Katic, Zlata Ozvacic, et al. 2008. "Burnout in European Family Doctors: The EGPRN Study." *Fam Pract* 25 (4): 245–65. doi: 10.1093/fampra/cmn038.

Song, Philip, and Rosalyn Stewart. 2012. "Reflective Writing in Medical Education." *Medical Teacher* 34 (11): 955–6.

Spears, Larry C. 1995. *Reflections on Leadership: How Robert K. Greenleaf's Theory of Servant-Leadership Influenced Today's Top Management Thinkers*. New York: Wiley.

Spector, Paul E., Zhiqing E. Zhou, and Xin Xuan Che. 2014. "Nurse Exposure to Physical and Nonphysical Violence, Bullying, and Sexual Harassment: A Quantitative Review." *Int J Nurs Stud* 51 (1): 72–84. doi: 10.1016/j.ijnurstu.2013.01.010.

Spivak, Gayatri Chakravorty. 1994. "Can the Subaltern Speak?" In *Colonial Discourse and Post-Colonial Theory. A Reader*, edited by Patrick Williams and Laura Chrisman, 66–111. New York: Columbia University Press.

Stergiopoulos, Erene, Rachel H. Ellaway, Nima Nahiddi, and Maria A. Martimianakis. 2019. "A Lexicon of Concepts of Humanistic Medicine: Exploring Different Meanings of Caring and Compassion at One Organization." *Academic Medicine: Journal of the Association of American Medical Colleges* 94 (7): 1019–26. doi: 10.1097/ACM.0000000000002732.

Stevens, Hallam. 2016. "From Medical Gaze to Statistical Person: Historical Reflections on Evidence-Based and Personalised Medicine." *Australian Family Physician* 45 (9): 632.

Street, Richard L., Lin Liu, Neil J. Farber, Yunan Chen, Alan Calvitti, Nadir Weibel, Mark T. Gabuzda, et al. 2017. "Keystrokes, Mouse Clicks, and Gazing at the Computer: How Physician Interaction with the EHR Affects Patient Participation." *Journal of General Internal Medicine*:1–6. doi: 10.1007/s11606-017-4228-2.

Stickley, Theo, and Dawn Freshwater. 2008. "Nursing Best Practice Guideline: Establishing Therapeutic Relationships." In *Learning about Mental Health Practice*, edited by Theo Stickley and Thurstine Basset, 439–61. Hoboken, NJ: John Wiley and Sons. doi: 10.1002/9780470699300.ch23.

Stroebe, Wolfgang, Margaret Stroebe, and Georgios Abakoumkin. 1996. "The Role of Loneliness and Social Support in Adjustment to Loss: A Test of Attachment versus Stress Theory." *Journal of Personality and Social Psychology* 70:1241–9.

Strudwick, Gillian. 2015. "Predicting Nurses' Use of Healthcare Technology Using the Technology Acceptance Model." *Computers, Informatics, Nursing* 33 (5): 189–98. doi: 10.1097/CIN.0000000000000142.

Strudwick, Gillian, Carrie Clark, Brittany McBride, Moshe Sakal, and Kamini Kalia. 2017. "Thank You for Asking: Exploring Patient Perceptions of Barcode Medication Administration Identification Practices in Inpatient Mental Health Settings." *International Journal of Medical Informatics* 105 (February): 31–7. doi: 10.1016/j.ijmedinf.2017.05.019.

Strudwick, Gillian, Carrie Clark, Marcos Sanches, and John Strauss. 2018. "Predictors of Mental Health Professionals' Perceptions of Patient Portals." *AMIA ... Annual Symposium proceedings / AMIA Symposium*, 989–97. AMIA Symposium.

Sunderji, Nadiya, Allison Crawford, and Marijana Jovanovic. 2015. "Telepsychiatry in Graduate Medical Education: A Narrative Review." *Academic Psychiatry* 39 (1): 55–62.

Susskind, Richard E., and Daniel Susskind. 2015. *The Future of the Professions: How Technology Will Transform the Work of Human Experts*. New York: Oxford University Press.

Tannenbaum, Cara, and Danielle Day. 2017. "Age and Sex in Drug Development and Testing for Adults." *Pharmacological Research* 121:83–93. doi: https://doi.org/10.1016/j.phrs.2017.04.027.

Taran, Shaurya. 2015. "Opinion: Student's Perspective of the Teaching of Empathy in Medical School." *Vancouver Sun*, 14 August 2015.

Terry, Christopher, and Jeff Cain. 2016. "The Emerging Issue of Digital
    Empathy." *American Journal of Pharmaceutical Education* 80 (4): 58.
Thomas, Larissa R., Jonathan A. Ripp, and Colin P. West. 2018. "Charter
    on Physician Well-being." *JAMA* 319 (15): 1541–2. doi: 10.1001/
    jama.2018.1331.
Tierney, Stephanie, Kate Seers, Elizabeth Tutton, and Joanne Reeve. 2017.
    "Enabling the Flow of Compassionate Care: A Grounded Theory
    Study." *BMC Health Services Research* 17 (174).
Timmermans, Stefan, and Rene Almeling. 2009. "Objectification,
    Standardization, and Commodification in Health Care: A Conceptual
    Readjustment." *Social Science & Medicine (1982)* 69 (1): 21–7.
    doi: 10.1016/j.socscimed.2009.04.020.
Topol, Eric. 2019a. *Deep Medicine: How Aritificial Intelligence Can Make
    Healthcare Human Again.* New York: Basic Books.
Topol, Eric. 2019b. *Preparing the Healthcare Workforce to Deliver the
    Digital Future.* NHS.
Trudeau, The Right Honourable Justin. 2018. "Canada's Vision for Global
    Health and Gender Equality." *Lancet* 391 (10131): 1651–53.
Trufelli, Damila. C., C.G. Bensi, J.B. Garcia, J.L. Narahara, M.N. Abrao,
    R.W. Diniz, C. Vanessa da Costa Miranda, Heloisa P. Soares, and Auro
    Del Giglio. 2008. "Burnout in Cancer Professionals: A Systematic
    Review and Meta-analysis." *Eur J Cancer Care (Engl)* 17 (6): 524–31.
    doi: 10.1111/j.1365-2354.2008.00927.x.
Turkel, Marian C. 2014. "Leading From the Heart: Caring, Love, Peace,
    and Values Guiding Leadership." *Nursing Science Quarterly* 27 (2):
    172–7. doi: 10.1177/0894318414522663.
UNAIDS (Joint United Nations Programme on HIV/AIDS). 2018. UNAIDS
    Data 2018. Geneva, Switzerland.
Valizadeh, Leila, Vahid Zamanzadeh, Belinda Dewar, Azad Rahmani, and
    Mansour Ghafourifard. 2018. "Nurse's Perceptions of Organisational
    Barriers to Delivering Compassionate Care: A Qualitative Study."
    Nursing Ethics 25 (5): 580–90.
Van Dierendonck, Dirk. 2011. "Servant Leadership: A Review and
    Synthesis." *Journal of Management* 37 (4): 1228–61. doi: 10.1177/
    0149206310380462.
Van Dierendonck, Dirk, and Kathleen Patterson. 2015. "Compassionate
    Love as a Cornerstone of Servant Leadership: An Integration of
    Previous Theorizing and Research." *Journal of Business Ethics* 128 (1):
    119–31. doi: 10.1007/s10551-014-2085-z.

Van Doorn, Yvonne, Joris van Ruysseveldt, Karen van Dam, Wilhelm Mistiaen, and Irina Nikolova. 2016. "Understanding Well-Being and Learning of Nigerian Nurses: A Job Demand Control Support Model Approach." *J Nurs Manag* 24 (7): 915–22. doi: 10.1111/jonm.12397.

Van Wynsberghe, Aimee. 2013. "Designing Robots for Care: Care Centered Value-Sensitive Design." *Science and Engineering Ethics* 19 (2): 407–33.

Varpio, Lara, Kathy Day, Pat Elliot-Miller, James W. King, Craig Kuziemsky, Avi Parush, Tyson Roffey, and Judy Rashotte. 2015. "The Impact of Adopting EHRS: How Losing Connectivity Affects Clinical Reasoning." *Medical Education* 49 (5): 476–86.

Virtanen, Marianna, Tuula Oksanen, Ichiro Kawachi, S.V. Subramanian, Marko Elovainio, Sakari Suominen, Anne Linna, et al. 2012. "Organizational Justice in Primary-Care Health Centers and Glycemic Control in Patients with Type 2 Diabetes." *Med Care* 50 (10): 831–5. doi: 10.1097/MLR.0b013e31825dd741.

Vogel, Lauren. "Canada Has a Long Way to go on Virtual Care." 2020. *CMAJ* 192 (9): E227–E228. doi: 10.1503/cmaj.1095851.

Wachter, Robert. 2015. *"The Digital Doctor": Hope, Hype and Harm at the Dawn of Medicine's Computer Age.* New York: McGraw-Hill Education, 2015.

Wallace, Jean E., Jane B. Lemaire, and William A. Ghali. 2009. "Physician Wellness: A Missing Quality Indicator." *Lancet* 374 (9702): 1714–21. doi: 10.1016/S0140-6736(09)61424-0.

Wartman, Steven A., and C. Donald Combs. 2018. "Medical Education Must Move from the Information Age to the Age of Artificial Intelligence." *Academic Medicine* 93 (8): 1107–9.

Wells, Helen. 1943. *Cherry Ames, Student Nurse.* New York: Grosset & Dunlap.

Wendsche, Johannes, Winfried Hacker, Jürgen Wegge, and Matthias Rudolf. 2016. "High Job Demands and Low Job Control Increase Nurses' Professional Leaving Intentions: The Role of Care Setting and Profit Orientation." *Res Nurs Health* 39 (5): 353–63. doi: 10.1002/nur.21729.

West, Colin P., Liselotte N. Dyrbye, Patricia J. Erwin, and Tait D. Shanafelt. 2016. "Interventions to Prevent and Reduce Physician Burnout: A Systematic Review and Meta-analysis." *Lancet* 388 (10057): 2272–81. doi: 10.1016/S0140-6736(16)31279-X.

232

West, Colin P., Tait D. Shanafelt, and Joseph C. Kolars. 2011. "Quality of Life, Burnout, Educational Debt, and Medical Knowledge among Internal Medicine Residents." *JAMA* 306 (9): 952–60. doi: 10.1001/jama.2011.1247.

West, Michael, and Rachna Chowla. 2017. *Compassionate: Concepts, Research and Applications, Compassionate Leadership for Compassionate Healthcare.* New York: Routledge/Taylor & Francis Group.

West, Michael, Regina Eckert, Ben Collins, and Rachna Chowla. 2017. *Caring to Change: How Compassionate Leadership Can Stimulate Compassion in Healthcare.* London: The King's Fund. http://tinyurl.com/lfykfl2.

Westermann, Claudia, Agnessa Kozak, Melanie Harling, and Albert Nienhaus. 2014. "Burnout Intervention Studies for Inpatient Elderly Care Nursing Staff: Systematic Literature Review." *Int J Nurs Stud* 51 (1): 63–71. doi: 10.1016/j.ijnurstu.2012.12.001.

Westley, Frances, Brenda Zimmerman, and Michael Quinn Patton. 2006. *Getting to Maybe: How the World Is Changed.* Toronto: Random House Canada.

Whitehead, Cynthia, Ayelet Kuper, Risa Freeman, Batya Grundland, and Fiona Webster. 2014. "Compassionate Care? A Critical Discourse Analysis of Accreditation Standards." *Medical Education* 48 (6): 632–43.

Whitney, Diana, Amanda Trosten-Bloom, and Kae Rader. 2010. *Appreciative Leadership: Focus on What works to Drive Winning Performance and Build a Thriving Organization.* New York: McGraw-Hill.

WHO (World Health Organization). 2010. *Framework for Action on Interprofessional Education & Collaborative Practice.* Switzerland: WHO.

Wikipedia. 2018. "Technology." https://en.wikipeida.org/wiki/Technology.

Wiljer, David, Rebecca Charow, Helen Costin, Lydia Sequeira, Melanie Anderson, Gillian Strudwick, Tim Tripp, and Allison Crawford. 2019. "Defining Compassion in the Digital Health Age: Protocol for a Scoping Review." *BMJ Open.* In press.

Williams, David R., Harold W. Neighbors, and James S. Jackson. 2003. "Racial/Ethnic Discrimination and Health: Findings From Community Studies." *American Journal of Public Health* 93 (2): 200–8. doi: 10.2105/AJPH.93.2.200.

Wilson, Kumanan. 2018. "Mobile Cell Phone Technology Puts the Future of Health Care in Our Hands." *CMAJ* 190 (13): E378–E379. doi: 10.1503/cmaj.180269.

Wisetborisut, Anawat, Chaisiri Angkurawaranon, Wichunda Jiraporncharoen, R. Uaphanthasath, and Phongtape Wiwatanadate.

2014. "Shift Work and Burnout among Health Care Workers." *Occup Med (Lond)* 64 (4): 279–86. doi: 10.1093/occmed/kqu009.

Women's College Hospital. 2018. "What Is the Health Gap and Why Should I Care?" http://www.thehealthgap.ca/.

Worline, Monica C., and Jane Dutton. 2017. *Awakening Compassion at Work*. Oakland, CA: Berrett-Koehler Publishers Inc.

Wozney, Lori. 2017. *Advancing the Evolution: Insights into the State of e-Mental Health Services in Canada*. doi: 10.13140/RG.2.2.21190.57920.

Wright, Alexi A., and Ingrid T. Katz. 2018. "Beyond Burnout – Redesigning Care to Restore Meaning and Sanity for Physicians." *The New England Journal of Medicine* 378 (4): 309–11. doi: 10.1056/NEJMp1716845.

Writing Working Group on behalf of the Indigenous Health Network. 2019. *Joint Commitment to Action on Indigenous Health*. http://www.afmc.ca/sites/default/files/pdf/AFMC_Position_Paper_JCAIH_EN.pdf.

Zamanzadeh, Vahid, Leila Valizadeh, Azad Rahmani, Margreet van der Cingel, and Mansour Ghafourifard. 2018. "Factors Facilitating Nurses to Deliver Compassionate Care: A Qualitative Study." *Scandinavian Journal of Caring Sciences* 32 (1): 92–97.

Contributors

JOCELYN BENNETT is a healthcare executive and nurse leader, and director of the Compassion Project at AMS Healthcare. She holds a lecturer appointment (status) with the Bloomberg Faculty of Nursing at the University of Toronto. Her expertise includes the design and evaluation of innovative models of care and environments to deliver the highest quality patient- and family-centred care.

MARION C.E. BRIGGS is an associate professor of clinical sciences at the Northern Ontario School of Medicine. A physiotherapist by profession, Marion's career has spanned forty-eight years in two countries (three provinces in Canada and two states in the USA). All of her postgraduate training and research have focused on organization and change in the context of collaborative practices in healthcare. As an AMS Phoenix Fellow, Marion developed a longitudinal postgraduate residency curriculum titled "Compassionate, collaborative, person-centred care."

DEANNA C. CHAUKOS is an assistant professor of psychiatry and associate director of the Psychiatry Residency Program at the University of Toronto. Her research focuses on medical education initiatives, including resident physician well-being and the impact of physician burnout on trainees.

ALLISON CRAWFORD is an associate professor in the Department of Psychiatry, the Dalla Lana School of Public Health, and the Department of English, University of Toronto. She is a clinician scientist and the associate chief of outreach and telemental health at the Centre for

Addiction and Mental Health, and co-chair of ECHO Ontario Mental Health. Her research interests centre around digital health equity, including person- and community-centred wellness.

CATHERINE CREEDE is a partner in the consulting firm The Potential Group, which focuses on designing and building capacity for sustainable strategy and change, primarily in the space of healthcare and education, within Ontario and across Canada. She is a consultant, educator, writer, coach, and leader with a mission to create sustainable, generative, socially accountable change. She has an adjunct faculty role with the Department of Psychiatry at the University of Toronto, and has been the volunteer co-director of a youth learning and development program in Uganda since 2007.

SANDRA FISMAN brings experiences from a generative career as a leader and administrator with concurrent clinical care practice for children, youth, and families. These perspectives have affirmed her philosophical premise that a compassionate organizational culture sets the sails for the patient-provider partnership. She has been involved with AMS Phoenix from its inception, chairing the Fellowship Advisory Committee.

BRIAN D. HODGES is professor in the Faculty of Medicine and the Ontario Institute for Studies in Education at the University of Toronto; executive vice-president education and chief medical officer at the University Health Network; and a practicing psychiatrist and teacher. His research focuses on assessment, competence, compassion, and the future of the health professions. His work has been recognized with the Association of American Medical Colleges Flexner Award (2015) and the Karolinska Institutet Prize for Research in Medical Education (2016).

JENNIFER JOHANNESEN is a parent whose son, Owen, had multiple severe disabilities all his life. He died in 2010 at the age of twelve. Her experiences as Owen's caregiver and advocate led her to ask broader questions about disability and society, special education, and clinical healthcare practice. Jennifer now writes, lectures, and consults on healthcare practice and policy related to patient-centred care, patient engagement, and critical thinking in clinical practice. She recently earned a master of science in bioethics from Clarkson University (Schenectady, NY) and is based in Guelph, Ontario.

RABIA KHAN is a PhD candidate at the Institute of Medical Sciences and the Collaborative Doctoral Program in Global Health at the Dalla Lana School of Public Health at the University of Toronto. Broadly, she is interested in the health of health workers. She investigates the phenomenon of burnout (at the level of trainees through to health systems), the globalization of medical education, and the intersection between global health research and health professions education.

ARNO K. KUMAGAI is professor and vice chair for education, Department of Medicine, University of Toronto Faculty of Medicine; researcher, the Wilson Centre, University Health Network; and the F.M. Hill Chair in Humanism Education, Department of Medicine, Women's College Hospital and the University of Toronto Faculty of Medicine. He has published extensively on the use of narratives in medical education, medical humanities, transformative learning, dialogical teaching, and teaching for equity and social justice.

AYELET KUPER is a physician with a doctorate in literature and a long-standing commitment to social justice. She is an associate professor and co-lead for person-centred care education in the Department of Medicine at the University of Toronto, a clinician in the Division of General Internal Medicine at Sunnybrook Health Sciences Centre, and a scientist and associate director at the Wilson Centre, University Health Network/University of Toronto. She was an AMS Phoenix Fellow in 2012–14 and currently sits on the AMS Phoenix Strategic Advisory Committee.

ANDREA LAWSON is the research lead in the Women's College Research Institute. She completed her PhD at the University of Western Ontario in social psychology, studying the perception of immigrants and immigration as a vector of disease transmission. She is an expert in project management and knowledge synthesis methodologies, and has conducted and co-authored several systematic and scoping reviews.

MANDY LOWE is the senior director, clinical education at the University Health Network and a strategic adviser for the Centre for Interprofessional Education at the University of Toronto. She holds a status appointment as assistant professor in the Department of Occupational Science and Occupational Therapy, Faculty of Medicine at the University of Toronto. Mandy is passionate about work that advances learning and caring through collaborative work at the interface of clinical practice, education, and research.

CLAIRE MALLETTE is an associate professor in the School of Nursing at York University. She has a diverse academic, research, and clinical background and has held leadership positions in both practice and academia. Her areas of interest and research are in compassionate care, technology, culture, and bullying in the workplace.

MARIA ATHINA (TINA) MARTIMIANAKIS is associate professor and director of medical education scholarship at the Department of Paediatrics, University of Toronto, and scientist and associate director, partnerships and collaborations at the Wilson Centre. She studies the impact of organizational cultures and structures on the socialization of health professional learners, the careers of clinical faculty, and the construction and performance of professional identities and expertise. As an AMS Phoenix Fellow and member of the AMS Phoenix Project Advisory Committee since its inception, she focuses on knowledge implementation to support compassionate organizational transformation and address conditions that impact the wellness of faculty and learners.

ROBERT G. MAUNDER is a professor of psychiatry at the University of Toronto and holds the Chair in Health and Behaviour at Sinai Health. His research focuses on childhood adversity and insecure attachment as determinants of health and the effects of stress on healthcare workers. He was the lead author on several publications documenting the psychological impact of the 2003 SARS outbreak on hospital workers.

THIRUSHA NAIDU trained and now practices as a clinical psychologist in South Africa. Her PhD was in psychology and health promotion. Her research focuses broadly on health humanities and medical education with an emphasis on health professionals' identity and reflective practice. Social equity, social justice, compassion, and empathy in healthcare – inspired by her work as a psychotherapist in resource-constrained settings in Africa – motivate and guide her research.

GAIL PAECH is the CEO of AMS Healthcare, which strives to improve the healthcare of all Canadians by innovating education and practice, championing the history of medicine and healthcare, supporting leadership development, and advancing research in the health humanities. Over her career, Gail has led in the public, private, and non-profit sectors, including senior management/CEO roles in hospitals and a global consulting company, as well as serving as associate deputy minister of economic development and trade and assistant deputy minister of health and long-term Care in Ontario. She is known for her leadership of large-scale projects focused on health system change.

KATHRYN PARKER is the senior director, academic affairs and the co-lead for the Centre for Leadership in Innovation at Holland Bloorview Kids Rehabilitation Hospital; associate professor in the Faculty of Medicine at the University of Toronto; and program evaluation consultant for the Centre for Interprofessional Education, University of Toronto. Her passion is to engage in collaborative work to move educational innovations forward within academic health science centres. She was the recipient of the 2013 AMS Phoenix Fellowship and was the recipient of the Larry Chester Award for Excellence in Strategic Leadership from the University of Toronto in 2013.

MORAG PATON is a PhD candidate in the Department of Leadership, Higher and Adult Education at the Ontario Institute for Studies in Education at the University of Toronto; a fellow at the Centre for Ambulatory Care Education, Women's College Hospital; and the education research coordinator in continuing professional development, PostMD Education in the Faculty of Medicine at the University of Toronto. Using a foundation of critical theory, her doctoral work explores the discursive construction of staff and faculty roles in health professions education.

LISA RICHARDSON is a clinician educator in the University of Toronto's Division of General Internal Medicine. Her academic interest lies in the integration of critical and Indigenous perspectives into medical education. She holds the roles of Strategic Adviser in Indigenous Health for the University of Toronto's Faculty of Medicine and for Women's College Hospital, and co-chairs the Indigenous health committee of the Royal College of Physicians and Surgeons of Canada.

DONALD ROSE is an associate professor at the Daphne Cockwell School of Nursing at Ryerson University. He has held several leadership positions in clinical practice, administration, and academia throughout his career. His research foci include compassionate care, technology, nursing ethics, and issues in forensic/mental health nursing.

PAULA ROWLAND is an assistant professor in the Department of Occupational Science and Occupational Therapy; cross-appointed faculty at the Institute of Health Policy, Management and Evaluation; and an education scientist at the Wilson Centre, all at the University of Toronto. As an AMS Phoenix Fellow, she studied practices of patient engagement, especially how organizations attempt to learn from patient and caregiver experiences in a continual effort to be compassionate places to give and receive healthcare. Her program of research continues to focus on questions of knowledge, power, and identity in connection with professional learning and organizational change.

JILL SHAVER is an independent consultant focusing on strategy development and implementation, organization and system change, and leadership development primarily within the public sector. She is co-director of the Collaborative Change Leadership Program at the University Health Network and is an adjunct faculty in the Master of Science in Organization Development Program at Pepperdine University in California.

MICHELLE SPADONI is an associate professor at Lakehead University School of Nursing. Her interests include nursing pedagogy that aims to support learners in rural and northern landscapes and exploring compassion in healthcare through artful and storied ways of knowing. Having lived in remote northern Manitoba as a child, and having Métis roots, she continues to evolve in her understanding of Indigenous philosophies. As an AMS Phoenix Fellow, she explores how healthcare practitioners are introduced to the meaning of reconciliation in relation to Canada's colonial past and present and how they understand Indigenous worldviews relative to their role, identity (personal and professional), and ways of being, doing, and knowing within the communities where they live and practice.

ERENE STERGIOPOULOS is a resident in psychiatry at the University of Toronto and holds an MA in the history and philosophy of science. Her research, conducted with Dr Tina Martimianakis, considers the experiences of medical trainees with disabilities, and the reframing of their patient experiences as sources of expertise for delivering compassionate healthcare. Her work has received funding from the AMS, and includes contributions to the AMS Phoenix lexicon project.

GILLIAN STRUDWICK is a scientist at the Centre for Addiction and Mental Health and an assistant professor at the Institute of Health Policy, Management and Evaluation at the University of Toronto. She is a 2018–2020 AMS Phoenix Fellow, and is currently the president of the Ontario Nursing Informatics Group.

MARIA TASSONE is the senior director, continuing education and professional development and co-director of the Collaborative Change Leadership Program, both at the University Health Network. She is the inaugural director of the University of Toronto Centre for Interprofessional Education and assistant professor in the Department of Physical Therapy, Faculty of Medicine at the University of Toronto. Her scholarly interests focus on leadership in complex systems, professional development, and knowledge translation in healthcare. Maria is most passionate about innovating at the interface of practice, education, and research.

DAVID WILJER is executive director of education, technology, and innovation at the University Health Network and an associate professor in the Departments of Psychiatry and Radiation Oncology, Faculty of Medicine, and the Institute of Health Policy Management and Evaluation, at the University of Toronto. His work explores the impact of digital technologies on the patient experience, patient engagement, and healthcare professional education and development, including co-creating digital technologies to promote high-quality, accessible, and compassionate care.

Index